Multiple Sclerosis
Fact Book

Multiple Sclerosis
Fact Book
Second Edition

Richard Lechtenberg, M.D.

Clinical Professor of Neurosciences
University of Medicine and Dentistry of New Jersey
Newark, New Jersey
Director, Professional Services
Berlex Laboratories
Richmond, California

 F. A. DAVIS COMPANY • **PHILADELPHIA**

F. A. Davis Company
1915 Arch Street
Philadelphia, PA 19103

Printed in the United States of America

Last digit indicates print number: 10 9 8 7 6 5 4 3 2 1

Medical Editor: Robert W. Reinhardt
Medical Developmental Editor: Bernice M. Wissler
Production Editor: Glenn L. Fechner
Cover Designer: Louis J. Forgione

Library of Congress Cataloging in Publication Data

Lechtenberg, Richard.
  Multiple sclerosis fact book / Richard Lechtenberg. — 2nd ed.
    p.   cm.
  Includes bibliographical references and index.
  ISBN 0-8036-0074-7 (pbk. : alk. paper)
  1. Multiple sclerosis.   I. Title.
  [DNLM: 1. Multiple Sclerosis.   WL 360 L459m 1995]
RC377.L43   1995
616.8'34—dc20
DNLM/DLC
for Library of Congress   94-25306
                                                       CIP

Dedicated to
Henry S. Schutta, M.D.

In appreciation for its significant contribution to continuing research and service to the MS community, the author has committed a percentage of royalties to the National Multiple Sclerosis Society.

Preface to the Second Edition

Since this book was first published, there have been several clinically important developments in multiple sclerosis research. For patients with relapsing-remitting multiple sclerosis, the most significant of these developments was the commercial introduction of interferon beta-1b (Betaseron), the first drug approved by the FDA specifically for the treatment of ambulatory patients with this form of multiple sclerosis. Studies using other interferons, including other beta interferons, are ongoing. Trials with Copolymer-1 (Cop-1) continue and should be completed in the near future. Innovative treatments, such as oral myelin basic protein and monoclonal antibodies, are being studied, and preliminary reports suggest that they hold promise. Unconventional treatments, such as beesting therapy, are greeted with muted skepticism. No one wants to deride a therapy until it has been conclusively dismissed in scientific studies. The current consensus is that several of the emerging approaches hold promise. After years of failing to influence the course of the illness, research is beginning to make inroads.

There is still no evidence that a cure is within reach, but further insights into the mechanisms of disease should lead to that ultimate goal. Better techniques for studying the disease, such as serial magnetic resonance imaging (MRI), should make it easier to recognize truly effective treatments when they do appear. Techniques for managing signs, symptoms, and complications of multiple sclerosis are being refined. Even though this disease still cannot be prevented or aborted, the quality of life for people with MS should continue to improve and the prospects for future innovations in treatment of the disease steadily brighten.

Richard Lechtenberg

Preface to the First Edition

Multiple sclerosis (MS) is a common disease that assumes many forms. Ideas on what causes it, what worsens it, and what will cure it have changed rapidly over the past few decades. Although no cure for multiple sclerosis has been found, many advances have been made in managing complications of the disease and in reducing the toll exacted by the disease. Much of what has been discovered about the disease and its management remains unavailable to people with the disease because it is in scientific books and journals. The language of science and medicine is a barrier between people with the disease and those investigating the disease. The principal objective of this book is to surmount that barrier.

This book presents and explains many of the current advances and controversies in multiple sclerosis. It provides information on the probable causes of, current management of, and evolving insights into multiple sclerosis in terms that nonphysicians can easily understand. This is a book for the person with multiple sclerosis and for those who care about that person. Practical solutions to the commonly faced sexual, social, and psychological dilemmas raised by the disease are considered in detail. The problems developing with medications, the potentials of therapy, and the promise of better approaches to this disease are also discussed.

This is a brief review of a topic that has expanded enormously over the past two decades, and so it is a selective review. Common approaches to the diagnosis of multiple sclerosis and practical aspects of managing the disease once it has been diagnosed are given much more attention than theoretical bases for the disease and the rationales behind research currently being done. A glossary of terms commonly arising in discussions of multiple sclerosis is included at the end of this book. For those interested in more theoretical and scientific discussions of various aspects of multiple sclerosis, there is also a list of recommended readings.

Richard Lechtenberg

Contents

What Is Multiple Sclerosis?

Multiple sclerosis (MS) is a disease of unknown cause that affects the nervous system. It may cause problems with vision, strength, coordination, speech, bladder control, sensation, or other faculties governed by the eyes, brain, or spinal cord. Both men and women are affected. The types of problems caused by this disease and the severity of those problems vary greatly from person to person. In any affected individual, the type and severity of problems associated with the disease are also likely to vary from year to year. How the disease will start, what course it will follow, and what chronic problems the affected person will acquire are unpredictable. Multiple sclerosis strikes people of most races and all social backgrounds, and it usually first appears in young adulthood. Because it is a relatively common disease and it affects individuals in what would ordinarily be their most productive years, multiple sclerosis has attracted considerable medical and social attention.

Basic Features of the Disease

Multiple sclerosis injures the **central nervous system** (Figure 1–1). The brain, the spinal cord, and closely related structures, such as

1

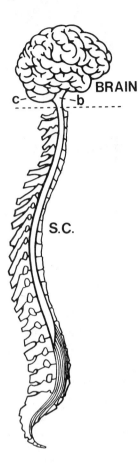

BRAIN

S.C.

FIGURE 1–1. *Central nervous system: The brain and spinal cord (S.C.) are the principal components of the central nervous system and are separated by a broken line in this schematic diagram. The cerebellum (c) and brain stem (b) are regions of the brain often affected by multiple sclerosis.*

the **optic nerves** to the eyes, are all part of the central nervous system (Figure 1–2). The nerves extending from the spine to the limbs, internal organs, and blood vessels are not part of the central nervous system and are not affected by this disease.

Within the central nervous system, nerve cells communicate with one another along fibers that cluster into bundles (Figure 1–3). **Nerve fibers** concerned with strength may run alongside other bundles concerned with pain perception, coordination, bladder control, or sexual function. These nerve-fiber bundles are the information-carrying pathways that are damaged in multiple sclerosis. Nerves to the limbs and internal organs, such as the

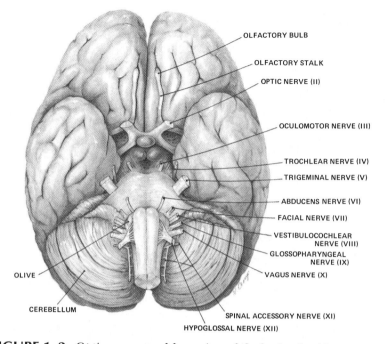

OLFACTORY BULB

OLFACTORY STALK

OPTIC NERVE (II)

OCULOMOTOR NERVE (III)

TROCHLEAR NERVE (IV)

TRIGEMINAL NERVE (V)

ABDUCENS NERVE (VI)

FACIAL NERVE (VII)

VESTIBULOCOCHLEAR NERVE (VIII)

GLOSSOPHARYNGEAL NERVE (IX)

VAGUS NERVE (X)

OLIVE

CEREBELLUM

SPINAL ACCESSORY NERVE (XI)

HYPOGLOSSAL NERVE (XII)

FIGURE 1–2. *Optic nerves and base view of the brain: Looking at the brain from below reveals numerous nerves and other structures not apparent from a side view. (Adapted from Gilman, S and Newman, SW: Manter and Gatz's Essentials of Clinical Neuroanatomy and Neurophysiology, ed 8. FA Davis, Philadelphia, 1992, p 9, with permission.)*

bladder and intestines, are not affected, but information pathways in the brain and spinal cord that connect to these **peripheral nerves** may be damaged. This damage in the central nervous system causes problems with strength, coordination, and sensation in the limbs and other structures that connect to the brain and spinal cord.

The name "multiple sclerosis" refers to two features of this disease (Table 1–1). The first feature is that *scattered* (that is, multiple) areas in the brain, spinal cord, and optic nerves are affected. Problems caused by the disease are also likely to be multiple, whether they are temporary or persistent. The second feature of the disease referred to in the name is the appearance

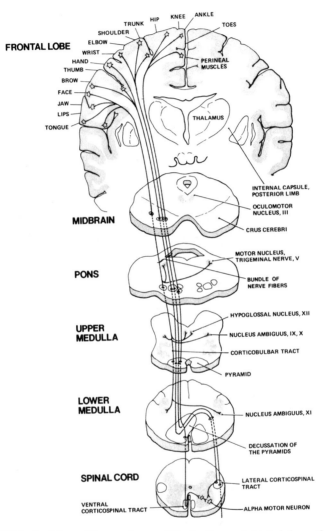

FIGURE 1–3. *Nerve fiber pathway: The pathway depicted from the brain to the spinal cord involves fibers responsible for control of movements. (Adapted from Gilman, S and Newman, SW: Manter and Gatz's Essentials of Clinical Neuroanatomy and Neurophysiology, ed 8. FA Davis, Philadelphia, 1992, p 77, with permission.)*

TABLE 1-1. Basic Features of Multiple Sclerosis

Disease involves the central nervous system.

Abnormalities are scattered about in multiple areas.

Plaques of altered nerve tissue develop.

Complaints involve unrelated elements of the central nervous system.

Complaints develop unpredictably at different times during adulthood.

No single test establishes the diagnosis.

The cause is not known.

No known cure exists.

There is no known prevention.

The disease has no significant effect on life expectancy.

---

of *sclerosed* (that is, hardened) patches in the involved areas of the brain and spinal cord. These sclerosed patches are called **plaques** and consist of nervous system tissue that has been altered by the disease. They are not necessarily regions of irreparable damage, but they do persist for years or decades in affected individuals.

A single plaque may extend across several nerve pathways. If it does, the person who has multiple sclerosis will abruptly develop problems involving several nervous system functions. Bladder problems and leg weakness may appear along with disturbed pain perception. If an individual plaque is very small, it may cause a fairly isolated disturbance, such as facial pain or double vision. Several small areas of disease may develop in the central nervous system at the same time, causing multiple but unrelated problems, such as disturbed vision, impaired sexual activity, and poor finger coordination. None of these problems, however, occurs only in people with multiple sclerosis. Other nervous system diseases, some of which are curable, can disturb the nerve pathways that are affected in multiple sclerosis, and so any individual developing these disorders must be investigated for reversible causes of the disturbed nerve function.

Who Has Multiple Sclerosis?

Establishing that someone truly has multiple sclerosis is neither simple nor foolproof, but an experienced neurologist, a physician specializing in the management of diseases of the nervous system, can usually decide if a person has the disease. The neurologist will consider the history of a person's problems, the problems revealed by physical examination of that person, and any information provided by laboratory tests. The extensive evaluation of the experienced physician is valuable in both establishing the diagnosis of multiple sclerosis and excluding other diagnoses. The complaints and problems that the physician routinely looks for are discussed in detail in Chapter 4.

No test or combination of tests allows a physician to state without question that an individual has multiple sclerosis. The changes in the nervous system, the plaques, that are typical of this disease are difficult to identify without actually dissecting the brain or spinal cord. That type of examination can be done only after the individual has died, and death is not the expected or usual outcome with multiple sclerosis. Imaging techniques that reveal the plaques, such as **magnetic resonance imaging** (MRI) or **nuclear magnetic resonance** (NMR) (see Chapter 5), are currently limited in the precision with which they allow identification of the lesions. No blood test has yet been developed that indicates plaques are present in the central nervous system.

How Certain Is the Diagnosis?

Because multiple sclerosis is not lethal, the presence of the disease must be determined with tests that neither invade nor injure the nervous system. The more commonly used tests are discussed in Chapter 5. Those currently available are usually adequate to establish the diagnosis soon after the first signs of disease appear, but in some cases the diagnosis must be inferred from the course of the illness.

The course of multiple sclerosis is quite variable. Because of this, many people are told by their physicians that they *possibly* or *probably* have the disease. The physician caring for an individual with typical signs and symptoms of multiple sclerosis usually will conclude that the person has *definite* multiple sclerosis only after several characteristic features have appeared and routine test results point to the diagnosis. "Possible," "probable," and "definite" are more than casual descriptive terms. They are levels of confidence in the diagnosis based on several criteria, including combinations of problems, patterns of recurrence, systems most impaired, and laboratory test results.

How Common Is Multiple Sclerosis?

The prevalence of multiple sclerosis varies from region to region, but in the northern United States and Europe, it is common enough to affect at least one relative, acquaintance, or colleague of almost every unaffected adult in the population. Precisely how many people are affected by the disease is unknown, but more than 1 in 1000 people in the United States carries the diagnosis. At any time, there are about 250,000 to 350,000 people with multiple sclerosis in the United States. The majority of these cases are in the northern states.

The true prevalence of the disease may be substantially higher than current estimates suggest. The reason for underdiagnosis is the absence of a foolproof test that will establish the diagnosis. Some physicians are reluctant to diagnose an individual as having multiple sclerosis because this is still viewed as a disabling and incurable disease. People with very mild cases are those most likely to be assigned other diagnoses, such as viral syndrome. If the disease progresses and typical signs of MS appear, the diagnosis will usually be revised.

Can It Be Prevented?

Multiple sclerosis cannot be predicted or prevented. Friends and relatives of an affected individual do not increase their risk of developing the disease by close contact with the affected individual. There is no evidence that the disease is transmitted from person to person. No diet, sanitary precaution, or exercise routine protects an individual against the disease or ensures that the disease will not get worse once it appears. This has not deterred a virtual army of concerned physicians, articulate patients, and outrageous quacks from formulating and publicizing countless recommendations and routines that are alleged to relieve or eradicate this **neurologic disease.**

Once multiple sclerosis is suspected, no strategy has proven effective against the progression of the disease. However, because so many people have this disease, almost any plan of treatment has its supporters. It is typical of multiple sclerosis that spontaneous improvement occurs. When this happens, the affected individual will quite naturally ascribe the improvement to the new item in his or her life. Simply expecting an approach to work increases the likelihood that the individual will believe that it has made a difference, a phenomenon called the **placebo effect.** Testimonials to miraculous cures do not alter the hard fact that currently there is no way to prevent or consistently affect the course of multiple sclerosis.

Can It Be Cured?

There is no known cure for multiple sclerosis, and it is unlikely that a cure will be discovered before the cause of multiple sclerosis is known. Ways to halt or reverse the disease are being sought through trial and error. This is not to say that progress has not been made in understanding and managing the disease. **Interferon beta-1b (Betaseron)** and Interferon beta-1a, synthetic proteins modeled after one produced by the human immune system, have spurred much discussion because of their ability to affect the course of the disease in some individuals with multiple sclerosis, but they are not a cure for multiple sclerosis (see Chapter 6).

The character and spectrum of multiple sclerosis are well known. The mechanisms involved in the appearance and progression of the disease have been explained in great detail (see Chapter 2). Probable causes for the disease are being investigated. Discovery of both the cause of multiple sclerosis and its cure is probably not far in the future; one or several of the research approaches discussed in Chapter 11 will probably lead to it.

How Does It Affect Life Expectancy?

Multiple sclerosis is not a lethal disease. As with any disease of variable severity, there are people who appear to have died as a consequence of an especially severe episode of disease, but this is exceedingly rare, and even then it is the result of a peculiar complication of the disease that is seen only in very young adults. Multiple sclerosis typically does not directly reduce a person's life expectancy. Complications of the disease, however, may result in a life span that is not as long as would be expected for individuals unaffected by the disease. In other words, if the multiple sclerosis is mild, life expectancy is not affected by it. If the disease causes numerous complications, such as recurrent skin ulcers, bladder infections, or pneumonia, life expectancy will be reduced to an extent determined by the complications that develop.

With the elimination of complications, a more normal life and life expectancy can be realized. Even for people with the most severe forms of the disease, the outlook has steadily improved during the past few decades. Improved management of infections and new techniques to reduce the risk of pressure sores have extended life expectancy and improved the quality of life for individuals with multiple sclerosis who have considerable paralysis and **spasticity.**

An essential part of reducing the risk of complications is regular follow-up care by a physician familiar with the patient and with the course and consequences of multiple sclerosis. Each person with multiple sclerosis has a unique set of problems that requires an individualized plan of action. The physician familiar with the patient can detect and manage problems with bladder function, skin care, depression, or sexual dysfunction before they become serious. The types of problems specifically monitored by the involved physician are discussed in Chapters 7 and 8.

Range of Severity

All discussions of multiple sclerosis are complicated by the variety of forms that the disease assumes (Table 1–2). The problems and concerns of the individual with mild visual loss associated with this disease are profoundly different from those of the person who cannot move the legs or has no bladder control. Both of these people may have multiple sclerosis, but to discuss their illnesses in the same terms is distressing for the one who is mildly impaired and inaccurate for the one who is severely impaired.

There is no level of disability that individuals with multiple

TABLE 1–2. Patterns of Disease

Course	Character	Frequency
Benign	Abrupt onset Few **exacerbations** (worsenings) No permanent disability	About 20%
Relapsing-remitting	Abrupt onset Periods of partial or total **remission** (improvement) Inactive for months or years	20%–30%
Relapsing-progressive	Abrupt onset Remissions initially Progressive disability later in course of disease	40%
Chronic-progressive	Slow onset of symptoms and disability Progressive problems and disability	10%–20%

sclerosis inevitably reach. If severe disability is going to occur, it usually develops within a few years of the first symptoms of the disease. The person who had a few mild episodes over the course of 3 years and then no attacks for 15 years should expect no additional problems caused by multiple sclerosis. Unfortunately, there are exceptions, and severe disease occasionally reappears after years of dormancy.

A physician familiar with the patient and with the disease can often adequately anticipate the problems the patient will face and help with long-term planning for the individual and his or her family. Rational approaches to the various problems that may develop with the multiple sclerosis are discussed in Chapters 7, 8, and 10. Strategies for modifying living arrangements to improve the quality of life are outlined in Chapter 9.

Physical Basis for Multiple Sclerosis

The human nervous system is a complex system composed of living cells that receive, transfer, interpret, and transmit information. Multiple sclerosis disrupts the communication among groups of these nerve cells, and as a consequence the operation of the nervous system is disturbed. Normal communication depends on connecting fibers that are very much like the wires in a telephone cable, each protected by its own coat of insulation. These connecting fibers are thin projections from the nerve cells and vary in length from fractions of an inch to feet (from microns to meters). The insulation around the connecting fiber is as vital to the transmission of information-carrying signals as is the fiber itself. In the brain, spinal cord, and nerves, this insulation is called **myelin** (Figure 2–1).

Myelin is literally wrapped around nerve fibers by the cells that produce it. In the brain and spinal cord, these insulation-generating cells are called **oligodendrocytes.** Hundreds or thousands of these myelin-producing cells line up along the nerve fiber to produce sufficient insulation for signal transmission along the fiber. Each oligodendrocyte produces a small patch of myelin

13

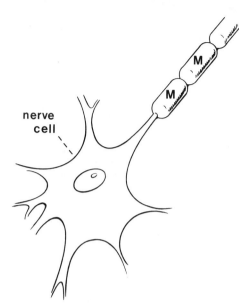

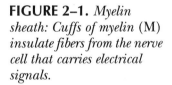

nerve
cell

FIGURE 2–1. *Myelin sheath: Cuffs of myelin (M) insulate fibers from the nerve cell that carries electrical signals.*

for each of several, adjacent nerve fibers. This process results in small patches of myelin along the entire length of the nerve fiber that abut, but do not fuse with, the myelin produced by other oligodendrocytes (Figure 2–2).

The advantage of the insulation is that it allows faster conduction of impulses along the nerve fiber, as well as better handling of closely spaced impulses. Nerve fibers covered with this myelin sheath of insulation are called *myelinated.*

In multiple sclerosis, the myelin sheaths in limited areas of the brain, spinal cord, or optic nerves are stripped off the nerve fibers they insulate. Bundles of nerve fibers lose their myelin protection over part of their length. When the myelin sheath is stripped away by any problem or disease, the nerve fibers are referred to as *demyelinated.* As mentioned in Chapter 1, pathways for different nervous system functions, such as vision, leg strength, and pain perception, are contained in distinct bundles of nerve fibers. The plaques of **demyelination** that occur in multiple sclerosis do not stop at the boundaries of these pathways, and so two or more pathways may be disturbed by a single plaque. The types of

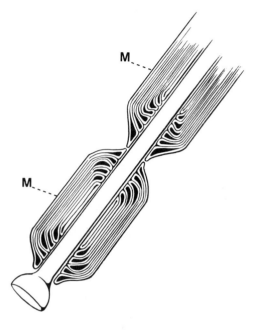

FIGURE 2–2. *Fine structure of the myelin sheath. Each section of the myelin sheath (M) consists of a many-layered coat of membranes that is stripped off during demyelination.*

problems a person will exhibit are determined by the pathways that are disrupted (Table 2–1).

In multiple sclerosis, the myelin is damaged or stripped off some of the nerve fibers; hence, MS is called a *demyelinating disease.* Other diseases can injure myelin and cause demyelination, but the causes and courses of these other demyelinating diseases are sufficiently distinct to allow no confusion with multiple sclerosis.

TABLE 2–1. Systems Often Affected

Vision

Coordination

Speech

Strength

Sensation

Bladder Control

Sexual Function

Demyelination does occur outside the brain, spinal cord, and optic nerves (the principal elements of the central nervous system) in other demyelinating diseases, but not in multiple sclerosis. Multiple sclerosis is the most common demyelinating disease of the central nervous system.

Demyelination is not the only change found in the nerve tissue of people with multiple sclerosis, but it is the principal change. Along with the damage to the myelin, there are signs of inflammation. Different types of white blood cells, called **lymphocytes,** and scavenger cells, called **macrophages,** collect in the areas where myelin is being damaged and appear to play a role in the demyelination process itself (Figure 2–3). Many of the changes in the brain and spinal cord are probably part of the recovery from each disease episode, but the cause and the consequences of the injury are still being argued.

Nervous System Damage

Each **flare-up** (*exacerbation*) of a person's symptoms is a sign that inflammation or demyelination is occurring. Inflammation, demyelination, or both may develop in several parts of the central nervous system at the same time, and wherever demyelination occurs, it produces the hard plaques of tissue, the sclerosis, that characterize multiple sclerosis. The agent or process initiating the attack on myelin in these plaques is unknown.

The symptoms produced are determined by where in the nervous system the demyelination occurs and how extensive it is. If demyelination occurs in the optic nerve, the person loses vision. If it occurs in the lower spinal cord, the affected individual may lose leg strength or bladder control. Many nervous system functions cannot be linked directly to a single bodily ability, such as vision or strength. Instead, some nervous system functions relate to less concrete traits, such as personality and mood, which also may be disturbed during flare-ups of the disease. Certain activities, such as vision and coordination, are affected more often than others, but which types of nervous system damage will occur in an affected individual is unpredictable.

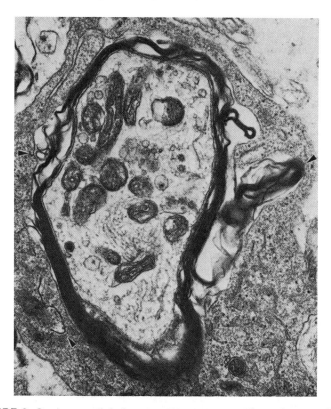

FIGURE 2–3. *A powerful electron microscope can show the actual destruction of myelin. Here, a partially demyelinated nerve fiber is surrounded by a macrophage. Some of the outer layers of the myelin have been loosened and are entering the macrophage (arrows). (From Prineas, JW: Pathology. In Cook, SD [ed]: Handbook of Multiple Sclerosis. Marcel Dekker, New York, 1990, p 209, with permission.)*

What Causes Multiple Sclerosis?

The cause of multiple sclerosis is unknown. Most current theories favor an infectious agent, such as a virus, but these are still just theories (Table 2–2). An alternative theory that has prompted much research over the past 20 years is that the immune system, the body's defense against infection, is defective or disturbed in

TABLE 2–2. Theoretical Bases

Infection

Autoimmune disease

Virus triggering autoimmune disorder

Virus disturbing immunity and allowing
    infection

people with multiple sclerosis. This deranged immune system either allows the central nervous system to be invaded by an agent that usually cannot get in or attacks the myelin sheaths of nerves as if they were foreign to the body.

Is It an Autoimmune Disease?

Many of the characteristics of multiple sclerosis suggest a disorder in which the body's immune system, which is designed to attack invading organisms such as bacteria and viruses, inappropriately attacks the body's own cells. This type of disorder is called an **autoimmune disease.** The theory that multiple sclerosis might be an autoimmune disease has directed much of the therapy aimed at this disease.

The evidence that multiple sclerosis is an autoimmune disease has always been open to question. In many autoimmune diseases, white blood cells produce proteins, called **antibodies,** that attach to the body elements under attack (Figure 2–4). Some investigators believe they have found antibodies that attack the oligodendrodocytes, the cells that make myelin, in the fluid surrounding the brain and spinal cord (*cerebrospinal fluid*) of people with multiple sclerosis. Such **autoantibodies**, as they are called because they attack the body's own cells, could explain many of the changes seen in the myelin, but it has not been proven that they actually produce disease. Even if autoantibodies that at-

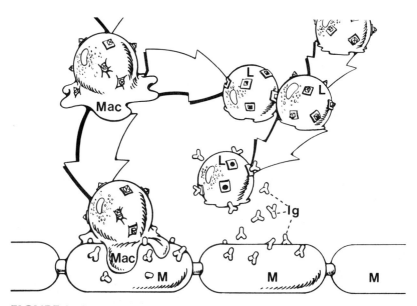

FIGURE 2–4. *Lymphocytes* (L) *and scavenger cells called macrophages* (Mac) *interact to produce antibodies* (Ig). *These antibodies and the macrophages seem to attack the myelin sheath* (M).

tack nervous system elements are found in multiple sclerosis, they may be consequences of an injury, rather than the cause of the injury.

The interactions between white blood cells and proteins in the blood, including antibodies, are very complex. Highly specialized cells (also called *killer cells*) are programmed to attack what are perceived as invading cells or organisms. If multiple sclerosis does result from disturbed functioning of the immune system, it may be these killer cells or other regulatory blood cells that are malfunctioning.

Even though the role of the immune system in multiple sclerosis has not been fully defined, many of the experimental therapies currently being tried assume that manipulation of the immune system can reduce the severity or frequency of demyelinating episodes. These experimental approaches are discussed in Chapters 6 and 11.

Is It a Viral Disease?

Many physicians believe that a virus plays a major role in the development of multiple sclerosis. This unidentified virus might be acting directly on the nervous system and injuring myelin or myelin-producing cells, or it may act much more indirectly. One indirect route would be for the virus to cause changes in the nervous system that elicit an autoimmune response. Autoimmune disease would cause the demyelination, but the autoimmune process would be touched off by the virus. Alternatively, the immune system itself could be injured by a viral infection, and an attack on the nervous system would arise with this injury. An even more complex hypothesis is that a viral infection disturbs immunity in a susceptible individual and that the disturbed immune system allows another virus to attack the nervous system. Many possible interactions between a viral disease and an immune problem can be imagined, but none has been established as the cause of multiple sclerosis.

There are several reasons to believe that an infectious agent, such as a virus, acts on the immune system to make an individual more susceptible to the disease or actually causes the disease. These include the low incidence of the disease in people growing up in certain geographic regions. In limited regions of the world, the disease has occurred in patterns typical of an epidemic, but no virus, bacterium, or other infectious agent has been convincingly linked to the disease in any of these areas. In fact, the most compelling argument against there being an infectious basis for multiple sclerosis is that after decades of research, no such basis has been found.

One infectious agent that has received considerable attention is the measles virus. Although the vast majority of people who have measles do not develop multiple sclerosis, there is a small group of individuals who report having had measles later in childhood than is usual, and this group shows an extremely high **incidence** of multiple sclerosis, but the measles virus has never been convincingly linked to the disease. That the measles virus or any virus is responsible directly or indirectly for this demyelinating disease remains to be proven.

What Makes It Worse?

The basic lesion in multiple sclerosis that causes worsening of signs and symptoms is the plaque of demyelination. As these plaques appear in different parts of the nervous system, new problems develop. The plaques may measure less than a millimeter or as much as a few centimeters (more than an inch) across; however, the location of the plaque is as important as its size. Widespread disease is likely to present more problems for the affected person than would a circumscribed disease, but a small plaque in a vital part of the brain or spinal cord can produce symptoms that are much more dramatic than those produced by a larger plaque elsewhere. In most individuals, plaques are widely distributed in the brain and spinal cord, and many of them produce no apparent problems. Obviously, a greater number of larger plaques increases the likelihood that the person will have signs of nervous system disease. As plaques accumulate or increase in size, nervous system function deteriorates.

New signs and symptoms may appear at any time, but there are circumstances that will predictably worsen a person's condition. A flare-up, related to an episode of demyelination in the central nervous system, may occur with or without provocation, but is certainly more likely to occur if the affected person's overall health is impaired. An individual with a cold or the flu is more likely to have a flare-up than one in good health. The problems that appear when the person with multiple sclerosis has an episode of worsening need not be new. Long-dormant problems with speech, coordination, bladder control, or strength may reappear when he or she has a viral or bacterial infection.

Even without such an episode, the symptoms of multiple sclerosis may worsen for a matter of minutes or hours in certain settings (Table 2–3). One such setting involves heat. A hot bath has an immediate and dramatic effect on the person's ability to function, but this effect is entirely reversible. Precisely why this occurs is not understood, but it is known that heat interferes with transmission of nerve signals along already impaired nerve fibers. The demyelinated fibers are less able to transmit information

TABLE 2–3. Causes of Temporary Deterioration

Heat

Hyperventilation

Dehydration

Sleep deprivation

Infections of any type

Medication effects

Anemia

Kidney disease

Liver disease

Other reversible organ disorders

when the affected person is in a hot environment. This deterioration occurs even without a change in body temperature; therefore, it is not a direct effect of warmer blood bathing the already impaired nerve fibers. What is clear is that the environmental stress of a warm bath or a hot room worsens the signs and symptoms of multiple sclerosis.

An equally brief worsening of neurologic problems will develop if the affected person hyperventilates (that is, breathes rapidly and deeply for several minutes). Hyperventilation changes the chemical composition of the blood only slightly, but the change is substantial enough to be reflected in the chemical composition of the fluid surrounding the brain. This transient chemical change interferes with normal brain and spinal cord activity in the person with multiple sclerosis.

Exhaustion, dehydration, and other causes of impaired resistance to disease also contribute to the temporary reappearance of dormant problems. People with multiple scherosis cannot tolerate prolonged sleeplessness or malnutrition. Such stresses invariably exacerbate the neurologic problems caused by multiple sclerosis. The manner in which each stress produces the deterioration may be quite distinct, but in each case the result is impaired signal transmission along marginally functioning nerve fibers.

Longer-lasting deterioration of nervous system function develops if the individual with multiple sclerosis has disease in a major organ, such as the liver or the kidney. Hepatitis, pancreatitis, kidney disease, and asthmatic attacks each place stress on the entire body. While these conditions are active, problems with walking, speech, vision, and other nervous system activities that seemed to have resolved long before may reappear. As the disease outside the nervous system resolves, the nervous system problems will improve.

What Makes it Better?

Improvement between flare-ups of multiple sclerosis may be complete or partial. There are probably several reasons why recovery occurs between attacks. To a small extent, some replacement of the injured myelin may occur. Probably more important are changes in the structure of the nerve fibers insulated by the damaged myelin. The fibers may not be as efficient in transmitting information without normal myelin, but they can change enough to accomplish this to at least a limited extent. Alternatively, other routes for handling information that do not involve the damaged pathways may develop.

Some recovery occurs because changes in the nerve tissue that appear with inflammation and demyelination resolve. One of these changes that interferes with nerve fiber activity is fluid retention in the brain and spinal cord. This fluid retention, called **edema,** may appear in the area of plaque formation and exert pressure on a much larger volume of nerve fibers than is actually demyelinated. As edema is eliminated from the central nervous system during the normal process of recovery, nervous system function improves.

If the myelin coat of the nerve fiber is replaced, the individual's symptoms should resolve. In mild cases, the resolution will be complete or nearly complete. If the nervous system fails to repair the damage or fails to develop an alternative method for getting information through or around the affected area, the attack will leave some permanent disability.

No diet, activity, or stimulus is known that will improve the nervous system's chances of recovering, but specific daily objectives and activities do seem to improve the outlook for early and prolonged recoveries from flare-ups (Table 2–4). As with any illness, a person should make every effort to follow a balanced diet and pursue reasonable activity. Excessive physical stress, such as crash diets and exercising until exhaustion, will slow the recovery after most illnesses, and multiple sclerosis is not an exception. Avoiding physical stress is definitely valuable, and many physicians believe that avoiding extreme emotional stress is also helpful.

Unfortunately, people may have little or no control over events that cause emotional stress, but they should pursue strategies that minimize chronic depression. Maximizing independent activity and maintaining a constant vigil for early signs of complications, such as the pain on urination that comes with bladder infections and the discoloration of skin in areas at risk for pressure sores, will also improve the outlook for long intervals free of disabling episodes. If complications are suspected, a physician should be consulted immediately, before the problem becomes substantial.

Many claims are made in the press and in private publications about effective approaches to multiple sclerosis, and most of these are nonsense. Electrical shocks to the nerves, acupuncture, chiropractic manipulation of the spine, and excessive vitamin intake at the time of a flare-up or between flare-ups will not improve the recovery achieved. The International Federation of Multiple Sclerosis Societies has compiled discussions of the more widely adver-

---

TABLE 2–4. Improving the Outlook

Maintain good nutrition
Continue appropriate activity
Avoid physical and emotional stress
Maximize independence
Watch for complications

TABLE 2–5. Prognosis

Nine out of ten people have long intervals with few or no symptoms.

One out of three has few or no symptoms for years after onset.

Three out of four are active and independent years after the diagnosis.

Lifespan is usually not shortened.

Flare-ups rarely occur after 45 years of age.

tised remedies in its *Therapeutic Claims in Multiple Sclerosis.* This and similar discussions listed in the Recommended Reading section of this book clarify the merit or lack of merit of therapies that are not specifically discussed here. The impact of beta interferon treatment on multiple sclerosis is discussed in Chapter 6.

The long-term outlook for the average person with multiple sclerosis is better than that for people with many other chronic diseases (Table 2–5), but the range of problems faced by individuals suffering from this disease is very broad. The prognosis (that is, the expected course and consequences of the disease) in 9 out of 10 cases is that the affected individual will have years of normal life disturbed by few or no symptoms of the disease. One third of all individuals will have few or no symptoms for years after the first episode of disease. Three quarters of affected individuals will have only relatively minor symptoms and can expect to be undisturbed by additional flare-ups of the disease after they are 45 years old.

What Is the Usual Course of the Disease?

Many different physical problems are produced by multiple sclerosis, but most occur with waxing and waning degrees of severity over the course of months, years, or decades. An individual problem, such as loss of vision or impaired strength, may appear abruptly, worsen over the course of days or weeks, and then improve over the course of weeks or months. Additional problems, such as slurred speech or unsteady walking, routinely develop in the same way. They may appear at the same time as the visual problem, weakness, or other initial symptom, or at a time when the initial problem is inactive.

Multiple sclerosis may cause a single episode of disturbed vision, repeated episodes of blindness, occasional bouts of difficulty with walking, or any of a hundred other transient or progressive disturbances or strength, sensation, vision, or coordination. Each time a symptom flares up, the person is said to have a *relapse,* or exacerbation. When the individual enters a period free of evolving symptoms, he or she is said to be in *remission.*

There are several different courses the disease may follow. If an individual has only one or a few episodes of abruptly appearing problems that resolve quickly and leave no permanent disabilities, the pattern of disease is called *benign.* About 1 out of 5 people with multiple sclerosis has this type of disease (see Table 1–2). If episodes of neurologic disease are more severe and occur more than a few times, but recovery from each episode is good or complete, the pattern is referred to as *relapsing-remitting.* If one problem after another appears with no apparent or significant respite from disease, the condition is referred to as *progressive* or *chronic progressive.* Some people with multiple sclerosis have remitting disease initially but develop progressive disease after years of relatively minor problems and are described as having *relapsing-progressive* disease. These progressive forms of multiple sclerosis account for about one half of all the cases identified, but even with progressive multiple sclerosis, the extent of difficulty faced by the individual varies from case to case. Men are more likely to have chronic progressive disease than are women. The basis for this sexual difference is unknown.

Most people with multiple sclerosis have distinct, isolated episodes of nervous system disease at some time in the course of the illness, but there are individuals who have few identifiable attacks. The disease may start insidiously and progress relentlessly, but this type of progressive multiple sclerosis is unusual.

The frequency, as well as the severity, of relapses is extremely variable. One person may have a relapse once every few years;

another may have severe flare-ups of the disease several times a year. As individuals get older they usually have relapses less frequently, but this may be of little consequence to one who was devastated by the disease before the age of 25. Teenagers with the disease are likely to have frequent relapses.

Terms such as "relapsing" and "remitting" are somewhat misleading because they suggest that multiple sclerosis is entirely inactive between obvious symptoms, and this is not so. Inapparent damage may occur in certain areas of the nervous system that will not cause immediate problems. If the parts of the brain that interpret subtle differences in melodies are injured, the person may never notice the problem unless he or she is a musician. Short-lived problems with sexual function or sleep may be dismissed as stress-related even if the individual consults a physician. If the progression between major flare-ups of disease is slight, that progression may be greatly overshadowed by the problems developing during the flare-up.

Who Gets Multiple Sclerosis?

Most people who get multiple sclerosis are young adults who live in a temperate, rather than a tropical, climate. No factors that make one individual more resistant than another to the disease have been discovered. Many factors have been thought to increase an individual's susceptibility to the disease, but few have withstood critical examination. These factors range from socioeconomic status to childhood illnesses. Concern that exposure to certain animals, such as pet dogs, increases the risk of the disease is still voiced by some physicians, but a strong connection between diseases carried by animals and multiple sclerosis has not been established.

The incidence of the disease suggests that if an infectious agent is responsible for multiple sclerosis, it produces symptoms in few of the people exposed to it, or it is not highly communicable. What is clear from population studies is that people are at risk for contracting the problem for only a few years of their lives and that the vulnerable age is at or near the time of puberty. Other factors increasing the likelihood that a person will develop multiple sclerosis include Scandinavian ancestry and a childhood spent in an economically developed country (Table 3–1).

29

TABLE 3–1. Likelihood of Getting Multiple Sclerosis

Greatest between the ages of 15 and 45

Greater for women than for men

Greater for people growing up in the temperate zones

Greater for specific ethnic groups, such as Scandinavians and their descendants

Greater for people living in developed countries with good sanitation

Greater for siblings and children of affected individuals

The Importance of Age

Most people developing multiple sclerosis are between 15 and 45 years of age. The disease may occur in people outside this age range, but illnesses resembling multiple sclerosis that occur in children younger than 15 years or adults older than 45 years are probably not multiple sclerosis. Diseases similar to multiple sclerosis occur at these ages, and some of these diseases are, in fact, demyelinating diseases of the nervous system; however, the demyelinating nature of these diseases alone does not mean they are multiple sclerosis.

Population studies suggest that most people who develop multiple sclerosis acquire the "cause" of the disease sometime between 10 and 15 years of age, that is, about the time of puberty (Table 3–2). The affected individual usually reports having lived at least 2 years in an area with other people diagnosed as having multiple sclerosis. This in no way suggests that multiple sclerosis is contracted from other people. Presumably, long exposure to agents in the environment places the child or young adult at risk for subsequently developing multiple sclerosis. Whether or not the disease will eventually appear in an exposed individual seems to be undetermined until at least 6 years after exposure to the responsible agent. This delay in disease acquisition has been calculated by studying people who have lived in areas with limited episodes of multiple sclerosis outbreaks.

TABLE 3–2. Hypothetical Timetable of Disease

Infancy	No disease
Puberty	Disease acquired but no symptoms
Young adult	Symptoms appear
Adult	Variable disabilities acquired, with remission or stabilization
Elderly adult	No new problems

To develop the disease eventually, people appear to require at least 4 years of exposure during the vulnerable puberty years in an area that has had many cases of multiple sclerosis over the course of several generations. This suggests that exposure to the agent responsible for multiple sclerosis during early childhood produces at least partial resistance in people subsequently affected (or infected). After acquiring the disease, symptoms will not appear for an average of 12 years. Even if the affected individual moves to an area free of multiple sclerosis, the disease will appear at 15 to 45 years of age. As discussed in the following section on the importance of geography, individuals who live until they are at least 15 years of age in areas that are not endemic for multiple sclerosis are at relatively little risk for developing the disease.

Differences Between Men and Women

Women are more likely to develop multiple sclerosis than men, regardless of the age of the individual (Table 3–3). At least 3 women suffer from multiple sclerosis for every 2 men affected by the disease, and in some regions the ratio is closer to 2 to 1. The basis for this difference is unknown.

Men with multiple sclerosis do not have milder forms of the disease than women, so it is not simply a matter of a greater tolerance of the disease. Men also develop the first symptoms of the disease at

TABLE 3–3. Sex Differences

Women affected 50% more often than men
Men symptomatic an average of 3 years later than women
Men more likely to get chronic progressive form
Severity of disease unrelated to sex

a slightly later age than women and are more likely than women to have the chronic progressive form of the disease. The average age at onset for women is 25 years, while that for men is 28 years.

For women, the disease is most likely to appear during the years characterized by sexual hormone activity essential for fertility. The disease invariably develops in women sometime between menarche, the onset of menstrual periods, and menopause, the cessation of menstrual periods. The significance of this is unknown.

Inheritance

The relatives of individuals with multiple sclerosis are often worried that the disease may be hereditary or may "run in the family." There is, in fact, a higher than expected incidence of multiple sclerosis in families with an affected member, but only the immediate family, the children, or the siblings of an affected individual are at significantly increased risk. If a parent has multiple sclerosis, the likelihood that one of his or her children will develop the disease is 15 to 20 times greater than that for other individuals in the general population. This is certainly something for people with multiple sclerosis to think about when starting a family, but the risk should not be overstated. Even with increased incidence in the children of affected individuals, the risk to these children is still only about 3 to 5 percent (3 to 5 out of 100).

Many factors contribute to the increased risk to offspring and siblings of affected individuals. Since the disease is not inherited and exposure to the affected individual plays no apparent role in the development of the disease, most physicians believe that what is shared in the family is a common susceptibility and a similar environment. Specific markers on many different types of cells, markers that are similar to those responsible for blood types, appear more often than would be expected by chance in people with multiple sclerosis. These characteristic markers are not responsible for the increased susceptibility, but they may be inherited along with other genetic factors that do increase the individual's vulnerability to the disease.

If resistance to the problem is low in one member of the family, it is likely to be low in others. Whatever causes multiple sclerosis is sufficiently widespread that all the members of a family living in the same area must be assumed to be exposed to it. Those who develop multiple sclerosis are those who do not have enough resistance to avoid developing it.

The more closely related individuals are, the more likely they are to face a similar risk of developing multiple sclerosis. Identical twins, that is, twins developing from a single fertilized egg, will both be affected by multiple sclerosis, if either develops the disease, in more than 3 out of 10 cases. Diagnostic tests, such as the MRI scan, which may demonstrate inapparent disease, suggest that risk to the identical twin of an affected individual is as high as 60 percent.

The risk facing the nonidentical twin of an individual with multiple sclerosis is much less than that facing the identical twin. Identical twins are 10 times more likely than nonidentical twins to both have multiple sclerosis if one is affected. The identical twins have identical genetic material, but both identical and nonidentical twins are as likely to have identical environments. This means that inheritance plays a significant role in determining whether or not someone will develop multiple sclerosis even though this is not a hereditary disease.

The Importance of Geography

Multiple sclerosis occurs much more commonly in certain regions of the world. It is common in Scandinavian countries and is more prevalent among people who have ancestors from Scandinavian countries. Where someone is living is obviously not the entire explanation for the individual's likelihood of developing multiple sclerosis, because even in Scandinavian countries there are ethnic groups, such as the Lapps, that exhibit a much lower incidence of the disease than their unrelated neighbors. Geographic location may be important if an individual already has a built-in vulnerability to the disease.

Looked at in terms of the incidence of the illness in different regions of the world, multiple sclerosis appears to be an acquired environmental disease. Waves of immigrants from areas with a high incidence of the disease to areas with previously few cases have produced dramatic changes in the previously unaffected areas. Looked at from a strictly epidemiologic viewpoint, it appears that an individual must live in a high-risk area for at least 2 years or be surrounded by people from a high-risk area for the same amount of time to acquire the disease.

Individuals growing up in tropical regions, such as equatorial Africa or South America, usually do not develop multiple sclerosis unless they move to a more temperate region, such as southern Canada, much of the United States, Europe, or Russia, before they complete puberty. A child leaving the tropics to live in the northeastern United States at 10 years of age may exhibit the same or nearly the same risk of developing multiple sclerosis as the child who spends all his or her youth in this temperate region. If that individual from the tropics lives in the tropics until the age of 17 or 18, the risk of developing multiple sclerosis is much less regardless of where he or she moves at that age.

Moves in the opposite directions at similar ages show similar patterns. The very young child acquires the risk of the area to which he or she moves. The young adult retains the risk typical of the area from which he or she moved. The disease or susceptibility to it seems to be acquired in childhood.

The rarity of the disease in tropical countries may be evidence of a lower prevalence of the causative agent in these areas, but there is also a genetic resistance to multiple sclerosis exhibited by populations originally from the tropics that is transmitted in the same way as other genetic traits. The young child from the tropics moving to a temperate climate may develop multiple sclerosis, but the risk is still less than that for the child whose ancestors lived in temperate climates. Temperate zones more remote from the equator are higher risk zones than those closer to the equator. This means that someone growing up in British Columbia, Canada, is at a higher risk for developing multiple sclerosis than is an individual living in New Mexico.

The importance of geography should not be overstated. Even in neighboring countries at the same latitude, the incidence of multiple sclerosis may be vastly different. In small countries with very different populations living near one another, such as Switzerland, the incidence of multiple sclerosis in these distinct communities may differ by as much as a factor of 6. This may reflect hereditary resistance to the cause of the disease rather than differences in exposure to the causative agents.

An equally reasonable explanation is that early exposure to numerous infections in the tropical and subtropical areas affects the immune system in some way that makes the individual more resistant to multiple sclerosis when he or she matures. Both the character of infectious agents in the tropics and the exposure to those agents would play a role in this explanation for the observed resistance to the disease exhibited by many of the people who have grown up in nontemperate areas.

How Does a Physician Diagnose Multiple Sclerosis?

Diagnosing multiple sclerosis is neither simple nor foolproof. There is no test that unequivocally proves that a person has the disease, and so some people are told they have some other disorder, or they are not given a diagnosis. This means that for many people the diagnosis is reached only after a long period of uncertainty. How long that uncertainty lasts depends more on the kinds of problems the disease causes in its first months or years than on the astuteness of the physician. When multiple sclerosis is finally proposed to explain the individual's complaints, the diagnosis is still just an opinion. If the physician making the diagnosis is a neurologist or other physician familiar with multiple sclerosis and similar diseases, that opinion will usually be correct.

Common Misconceptions

Most people first told that they have multiple sclerosis do not understand what that means. If they have known people with severe disease, they often incorrectly assume that they will neces-

37

sarily develop the same problems. This common misconception is both distressing and demoralizing. That many people with the disease have no disabilities is unappreciated because people with mild disease usually do not reveal to friends and coworkers that they have multiple sclerosis. Statistics on the probable course of the disease are too impersonal to provide much comfort to the individual with the illness. The actual course the disease will take is uncertain, and that uncertainty is a legitimate source of concern. What the affected person should recognize is that the course of the disease often is not severe.

Uncertainty of the Diagnosis

Adding to the concern aroused by the diagnosis of multiple sclerosis is the uncertainty of the diagnosis. With any disease, the diagnosis is simply the physician's leading suspicion. In multiple sclerosis more than most diseases, it is truly a best guess. It is a guess based on what the individual has experienced in the past, the history of the disease; what he or she currently complains of, the symptoms of the disease; what the physician finds on physical examination, the signs of the disease; and what is revealed by various laboratory tests, the diagnostic studies. This does not mean that the diagnosis cannot be made with confidence. In fact, a diagnosis of multiple sclerosis reached by an experienced physician on the basis of strictly clinical information, such as signs, symptoms, and disease course, will be accurate at least 95 percent of the time. In most cases, the person's history, signs, symptoms, and diagnostic test results overwhelmingly suggest multiple sclerosis before the diagnosis is reached.

There are, however, several diseases that can produce symptoms similar to those appearing with multiple sclerosis. That someone has poor vision with pain in the eye does not mean that he or she has multiple sclerosis. In fact, that type of problem is more likely to be a sign of glaucoma, a disturbance in pressure within the eye, than of multiple sclerosis. Decreased pain perception may develop because of a pinched nerve. Poor bladder control may be traced to a urinary tract infection. Slurred speech may indicate an injury to the coordination center of the brain, the **cerebellum,** or intoxication with illicit or prescribed drugs. Unsteadiness in walking can develop because of joint, muscle, or nerve disease. Combinations of these signs and symptoms will develop with a variety of central nervous system diseases unrelated to multiple sclerosis. Some of these can be cured and many can be treated. Early after the diagnosis of multiple sclerosis is reached, that diagnosis must be subject to reconsideration until the course of the affected individual's signs and symptoms makes the diagnosis certain.

The History

What is most typical of multiple sclerosis is its course. However, the course or history of any disease can only be studied by reviewing how the disease has developed and observing how it evolves. It is only after the person has had several problems, such as visual loss, fatigue, and bladder problems, that the diagnosis of multiple sclerosis can be made with confidence. It is not reasonable to expect a secure diagnosis of multiple sclerosis to be made in fewer than 3 months after the appearance of the first symptom, and it is much more routine for a diagnosis of multiple sclerosis to be established only after a year or two following the first symptom.

Any time neurologic problems appear, the affected person should consult a physician experienced in dealing with neurologic diseases and allow him or her to decide what the significance of the problem is. The physician will review the person's history, consider each of the current symptoms, perform a physical examination, and proceed with diagnostic tests that will help establish the proper diagnosis. The types of problems that commonly develop with multiple sclerosis are discussed below, along with the significance of a few of the many physical signs that develop with the disease. Diagnostic tests are discussed in Chapter 5.

The Symptoms

Symptoms by definition are the problems that patients complain of. Certain complaints in combination are heard more often with multiple sclerosis than with other diseases. Problems with vision, speech, walking, coordination, and urination are often reported by people who have multiple sclerosis (Table 4–1). When several of these symptoms develop at different times over the course of months or years, the diagnosis of multiple sclerosis becomes more likely.

What is most important in considering the significance of any symptom is the context in which it appears (Table 4–2). The abrupt loss of vision a few months after an unexplained episode of staggering or of slurred speech is very suggestive of multiple sclerosis. Weakness and numbness in both legs with poor bladder control and a history of unexplained visual loss is, again, a series of problems that suggests multiple sclerosis.

TABLE 4–1. Common Symptoms of Multiple Sclerosis

Blurred or double vision
Loss of vision in one eye
Slurred or slowed speech
Easy fatigability
Psychologic changes
Weakness or paralysis of limbs
Poor coordination
Shaking of limb
Staggering
Poor balance
Dragging feet
Numbness or pins and needles
Poor bladder or bowel control

TABLE 4–2. Pattern of Symptoms

Vary greatly from person to person
Vary over time in each individual affected
First symptoms usually in young adults
Early symptoms are usually temporary
Early symptoms usually include problems
   with vision
Problems develop in more than one nervous-
   system function
Acute symptoms are usually followed by
   months or years free of apparent disease

Visual Problems

With inflammation of the optic nerve, the person with multiple sclerosis will have temporary loss or disturbance of vision. The optic nerve is structurally part of the brain rather than a true nerve, so that, like the remainder of the central nervous system, it is susceptible to injury from demyelinating disease. Inflammation of the optic nerve is called **optic neuritis,** and it is an especially common problem in multiple sclerosis. Infections and metabolic (that is, chemical) problems can also cause optic neuritis in young people, but a great many young people who develop optic neuritis (more than 90 percent in some countries) prove later to have multiple sclerosis.

Vision may blur over the course of minutes or hours, and total loss of vision is common when optic neuritis first develops. Vision returns partially or fully within days or weeks if the problem is optic neuritis. One eye at a time is usually affected, but both eyes routinely will be affected by optic neuritis at some time in the course of multiple sclerosis. Changes in the nerve may be so subtle that the patient is never aware of the inflammation in one of the eyes even if both eyes are affected. In some people, vision problems will persist; in some, the impairment of vision is very slight, but in others it may be substantial. Complete, unchanging blindness does not typically develop with multiple sclerosis.

Color vision is especially vulnerable to demyelinating disease simply because it is a fairly restricted part of vision that requires a great many fibers from the eye to accurately transmit the information that is interpreted by the brain as color. A plaque of demyelination in the optic nerve need only damage a fraction of the total fibers carrying information on color to disrupt color perception. The high-resolution area of central vision accounts for most color perception, so an injury that affects the nerve fibers from these high-resolution light sensors will affect color vision.

Normal vision includes a small blind spot that is off to the side from central vision in both eyes. All of the nerve fibers from the membrane of light sensors in the eye, the retina, exit at the same point on the back of the eye, and at that exit point, called the *optic disc,* there are no light sensors. Any image falling on the optic disc will not be seen. Because this is a relatively small area in a part of the field of vision that produces low-resolution images, it is unnoticed by the normal person. With recurrent optic neuritis, however, this blind spot may enlarge and produce a much larger blind spot, called a **centrocecal scotoma,** which affects the area of central vision (Figure 4–1). Any blind spot that extends across central vision, where visual acuity is greatest, will interfere substantially with sight.

Abnormal Speech

Changes in speech occasionally develop in people with multiple sclerosis. The most common of these changes is slowing of speech and slurring of words. The other common alterations in speech involve changes in rhythm. The fundamental disturbance is in coordinating the movement of the tongue, lips, palate, vocal cords, and other elements vital to normal speech. Problems with the clarity or rhythm of speech are called **dysarthria.**

With severe dysarthria, the affected individual may exhibit a lilting or sing-song quality to speech that is called **scanning.** The rhythm of speech is inappropriate, and the person seems to exaggerate the natural rhythm with stops and starts in clearly inappropriate places. Speech is labored and does not sound spontaneous or lyrical.

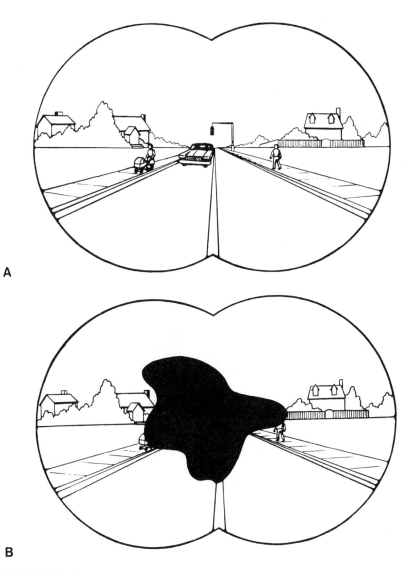

A

B

FIGURE 4–1. *Centrocecal scotoma:* (A) *Acuity is best in the center of a normal visual field.* (B) *With a centrocecal scotoma, central vision is lost and the individual must rely on peripheral vision.*

The part of the brain responsible for coordinating many types of movements is called the cerebellum. Speech is often disturbed in multiple sclerosis because the cerebellum is especially likely to be damaged in this disease. Some individuals with severe dysarthria are unaware that their speech is abnormal, but most will complain that their speech is more labored. If they are aware of the speech difficulty, speech therapy may help improve the clarity of the affected individual's language.

Fatigue

Loss of energy, persistent fatigue, and limited tolerance of exercise are common complaints in people with multiple sclerosis. Pervasive fatigue, however, is not limited to this type of nervous system disease and in fact may not even indicate disease of the nervous system. Chronic infection, diabetes mellitus, thyroid disease, heart failure, kidney disease, and dozens of other chronic problems can cause the same easy fatigability. What is distinctive in the person with multiple sclerosis is that the lack of energy cannot be explained by any of these other medical problems.

Depression can also cause easy fatigability and malaise, but that an individual is depressed does not necessarily explain the symptom of fatigue. With chronic fatigue, many people become depressed. The symptom is the cause of the psychologic problem, rather than the psychologic problem being the cause of the symptom. Indeed, people with multiple sclerosis may be easily fatigued and severely depressed as separate manifestations of their disease.

Psychologic Changes

Changes in personality and mood are common with many chronic illnesses, but in multiple sclerosis these changes may appear independently of other signs. Depression may be a major problem even when the affected person is not significantly disabled by the neurologic disease. It is again the course of the disorder and the associated problems that should suggest multiple sclerosis. A young woman who becomes severely depressed or inappropriately euphoric after a bout of visual loss caused by optic neuritis should be evaluated for possible multiple sclerosis.

With this disease, more than with other chronic illnesses, the problems with diagnosis and the vagueness of symptoms may lead family members and physicians to suspect that many of the patient's problems are imaginary. If psychologic problems or problems with recall appear, it becomes even more probable that the patient's symptoms will be dismissed as delusions. Family members and friends often cling to this notion even after the diagnosis of neurologic disease has been made, because it is less worrisome to dismiss a loved one's problems as psychologic than it is to recognize them as a consequence of nervous system disease.

In some families there is a concerted effort to hide the diagnosis from the affected person, who is told that he or she is imagining trouble. This approach is ill-advised because it leaves the person feeling impaired and confused. The truth usually surfaces despite all efforts to suppress it, and when that happens, the person loses trust in other family members. These and other problems developing because of the psychologic disturbances occurring with multiple sclerosis are discussed in detail in Chapter 8.

Difficulty with Walking and Coordination

Problems with coordination are common and are usually not from demyelinating disease, but when a young adult abruptly develops clumsiness or difficulty in walking, multiple sclerosis is one of the causes that must be considered. The coordination problem may actually prove to be from weakness or loss of normal sensation, but many individuals with multiple sclerosis have no loss of strength or sensation although they exhibit substantial problems in manipulating small objects and in walking.

Walking difficulty may be attributed to dizziness, that is, a feeling of postural unsteadiness, but usually it arises from problems with coordinating limb movements, called **ataxia.** Damage to the part of the brain most responsible for posture, the cerebellum, causes problems with directing limb movements individually and in concert. This means that an affected individual may be able to move each arm or leg fairly smoothly, but be unable to walk without staggering or unable to manipulate objects in both hands without dropping them.

Dizziness is also fairly common with a flare-up of multiple sclerosis, but **vertigo** is not. Vertigo involves the illusion of movement; the room actually appears to spin or the person affected feels himself or herself spinning. Vertigo is more likely to develop with a problem in the ear than with a problem in the brain or **brain stem.**

In its most extreme manifestation, the person with coordination problems may stagger when trying to walk (**gait ataxia**), fall when trying to stand, or scribble unintelligibly when trying to write. This degree of incoordination or clumsiness is not likely early in the course of multiple sclerosis, but severe episodes of incoordination may appear and then improve during the course of the illness. After several episodes of demyelination, some of the clumsiness usually persists.

Even complete loss of coordination in a limb does not indicate that a long-term problem with coordination will persist. Very fine coordination, such as that required for playing a musical instrument, may be lost, but the coordination required for writing and walking will usually return after the episode. People with severe disease may develop such profound clumsiness that they are unable to dress or feed themselves, but this is unusual.

Altered Sensations

There are numerous ways in which sensations may be altered (Table 4–3). Many people expect that with nervous system damage the most common complaint will be **anesthesia,** that is, complete loss of all feeling, over any affected skin surface. In fact, loss of feeling occurs much less often than do changes in feeling. A large patch of skin may tingle or burn for days or weeks. The soles of the feet may feel wooden. Light pressure over an area insensitive to pinprick may produce severe pain. These limited areas of altered sensation are called **focal deficits.**

TABLE 4–3. Types of Abnormal Sensation

Anesthesia	Loss of all pain, touch, and temperature sense
Paresthesia	Pins-and-needles sensation
Hyperpathia	Increased sensitivity to pain
Dysesthesia	Pain produced by a nonpainful stimulus

Altered sensations of any type develop with many different diseases affecting the nerves to the skin, as well as with those disturbing the pathways transmitting sensory information in the spinal cord and brain. Diabetes mellitus, vitamin deficiency, and poisoning are the most common chemical causes of sensory problems. When a nerve is crushed by superficial pressure, such as from poorly fitting boots, overly tight shoes, or improperly fitted girdles, the pattern of disturbed feeling will indicate that a peripheral nerve, not a central nervous system pathway, has been damaged. Peripheral nerve damage is not characteristic of multiple sclerosis.

If disturbed sensation occurs without any other neurologic problems, it is usually not from multiple sclerosis. If it occurs along with episodes of blindness, loss of bladder control, or slurred speech, it may well be a symptom of multiple sclerosis. The symptom of altered sensation cannot be considered separately from the individual's other complaints.

Decreased Feeling

A wide variety of changes in sensation are possible with multiple sclerosis. These range from pins-and-needles sensations to extreme sensitivity to touch. The pins-and-needles or tingling sensations over relatively insensitive areas are called **paresthesias.** Painful alterations of touch and pressure perception are called

dysesthesias. When a patch of skin is uncomfortably sensitive to minor stimuli, the disturbance is called **hyperpathia.** Of course, it is also possible to lose all sensation over some of the skin, but this absence of feeling (anesthesia) is not at all likely with demyelinating disease. Paresthesias, hyperpathia, and dysesthesias are all common in people with multiple sclerosis.

Chronic Pain

An individual with multiple sclerosis may be plagued by chronic pain for one of several reasons. It occasionally arises as a direct consequence of the demyelination in the central nervous system, but just as often—if not more often—it is a complication of the nervous system disease, a complication of treatment, or a sign of a local disease that has been masked by the multiple sclerosis.

The brain has no pain fibers to itself, so no amount of brain injury will produce pain. A tumor or inflammation in the brain causes pain by stretching pain receptors on superficial blood vessels or by stretching certain parts of the covering of the brain, the meninges. However, the systems that register and analyze pain information from all over the body are systems in the brain, and injury to these nerve groups can produce *illusory pain* (that is, pain that seems to originate in another part of the body, even though there has been no actual damage to that body part). Substantial damage to pain-processing centers in the brain can produce chronic discomfort. This disturbed perception may be limited to one part of the face or may extend over an entire side of the body.

Acute Pain

Whenever pain develops over a limited area of the body, the patient and physician should carefully examine the area involved to look for an unsuspected infection or injury. An abscess developing deep in tissues under an area that is repeatedly injured may reveal itself as an area of point tenderness with swelling and firmness of the infected tissues. If a ligament in a joint or the tendon of a muscle is strained or bruised, there may be pain that occurs only when the affected limb is in certain positions. With poor coordination or simply as a consequence of weakness, joints may suffer traumatic injuries. The treatment for these types of pain is management of the underlying infection or injury.

Fractures or dislocations of bones may occur in people with multiple sclerosis because weakness has allowed abnormal strains on joints and bones or because steroid therapy, a common treatment approach during flare-ups of multiple sclerosis, has weakened the intrinsic structure of the bone. An especially common complication of steroid treatment is the vertebral fracture. In this type of injury, the body of the spinal bone collapses on itself in what is called a *compression fracture.* This may be extremely painful and yet produce no problems other than the pain. The weight of the trunk usually drives the bony elements into each other. This type of fracture is usually seen at the level of the mid or low back. Again, management of the pain, as discussed in Chapter 7, must involve treatment of the underlying problem.

The person with multiple sclerosis is also at risk for developing acute pain problems because of disturbed muscle activity. Forceful contractions of the muscles because of involuntary spasms are often very painful. Slight changes in strength and coordination will place inappropriate stresses on joints, and arthritis may develop. This is especially likely with weakness in a leg. The ankle, knee, or hip joints may be damaged by improper alignment of the leg in walking. With injury to these joints, the spine routinely develops joint damage and the pain spreads to the back.

Persistent, forceful muscle spasms will fix the legs and arms in abnormal postures and produce *contractures* (shortening and distortion) of tendons. These contractures interfere with movement. Attempts at moving an arm or leg affected by such spasms can cause a great deal of pain. This problem affects only the most severely disabled individuals, but even those much less impaired may have similar pain problems. Relatively slight limitations of movement may force the limbs into abnormal positions that are painful in themselves. Physical therapy, as discussed in Chapter 10, is often very successful in relieving the chronic pain that arises with disturbed limb movements.

Facial Pain

Pain in the face is a relatively common problem with multiple sclerosis. It has several potential causes. Local infection or injury is always likely, but if this has been eliminated as a possibility by careful examination and radiologic studies, an injury to nervous system pathways must be considered. With damage to brain-stem pain pathways, the person with multiple sclerosis may develop an extremely uncomfortable facial sensation called **trigeminal neuralgia** or **tic douloureux** (Figure 4–2).

With this neuralgia, the individual has shock-like spasms of pain that seem to originate from a relatively small area on the face. Chewing, brushing teeth, shaving, or just touching a small patch of skin may trigger the sharp bursts of pain. Although this is one of the most severe pains likely to torment a person with multiple sclerosis, it is one of the most treatable. The various medical and surgical options useful for trigeminal neuralgia are discussed in Chapter 7.

Eye Pain

With optic neuritis there is usually pain in or behind the eye associated with the loss of vision. This type of pain may be worsened by eye movements, but it usually persists even when the eye is still. Although it is invariably temporary, the severity of the pain may justify treatment even if the severity of visual loss does not. With this type of pain, just as with every other type of pain, the affected person should consult a physician to establish that there is no treatable disease, such as glaucoma, responsible for the symptom. Techniques for managing the pain of optic neuritis are discussed in Chapter 7.

Bladder Disturbances

Bladder disturbances that may develop with multiple sclerosis include being unable to urinate when inclined to and being unable to prevent bladder emptying when it is inappropriate. If an

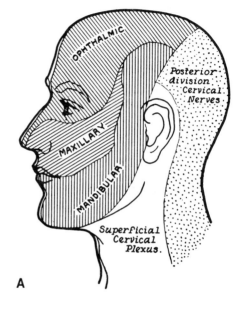

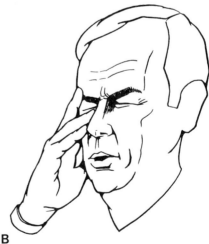

FIGURE 4–2. (A) *The areas of the face are supplied by the three principal divisions of the trigeminal nerve (ophthalmic, maxillary, and mandibular). (B) Shooting facial pains are characteristic of trigeminal neuralgia. (A, From Mancall, EL: Alpers and Mancall's Essentials of the Neurologic Examination, ed 2. FA Davis, Philadelphia, 1981, p 67, with permission.)*

individual has difficulty in emptying the bladder, the problem is called **urinary retention.** If premature emptying occurs, it is called **incontinence.** Many individuals with multiple sclerosis have some control over bladder emptying, but the degree of control is inadequate. They have an abrupt urge to urinate, and unless they urinate within seconds or minutes, the bladder empties involuntarily. This feeling that there in an immediate need to urinate is called *urgency.* All these complaints develop because the spinal cord pathways to the bladder are disturbed by the demyelinating disease (Figure 4–3).

The bladder is controlled by complex nervous system pathways that work in opposition to one another. Much of the machinery managing bladder emptying is handled by a system called the *sympathetic* nervous system; the machinery responsible for inhibiting bladder emptying is controlled largely by the *parasympathetic* nervous system. Many drugs are available that will influence either the sympathetic or parasympathetic systems alone, so pharmacologic control of the bladder may be achieved, as discussed in Chapter 7, even if nervous system disease has disrupted voluntary bladder control. Unfortunately, the sympathetic and parasympathetic systems control other organs besides the bladder, and the drugs that act on the bladder affect other organs. These drugs produce side effects in organs ranging from the intestines to the salivary glands, and so their usefulness is often limited by their unwanted effects.

Any adult under 30 years of age who develops problems with controlling the urinary bladder must be investigated for multiple sclerosis unless local damage or infection is evident on examination of the bladder. If multiple sclerosis is going to cause a problem with bladder control, the problem will usually be retention, rather than leaking, of urine. Even though retention is the underlying problem, a person's first complaint is often urgency, the need to urinate immediately, or incontinence, the inability to prevent the accidental loss of urine.

With urgency, the bladder must be emptied within minutes or seconds or incontinence will occur. It is not an illusion that the bladder must be emptied quickly. As the urgency worsens,

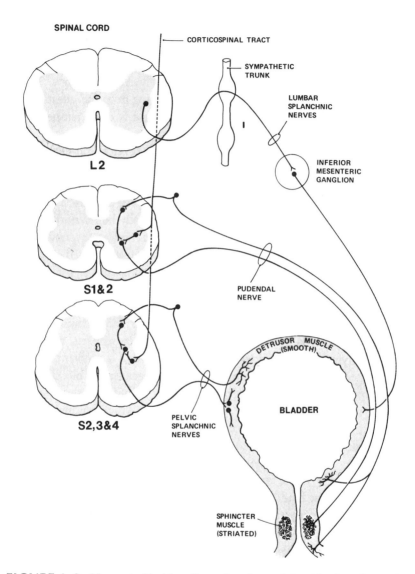

FIGURE 4–3. *Nerves to bladder: Several regions of the spinal cord supply nerves to the muscular wall of the urinary bladder to control bladder emptying. (Adapted from Gilman, S and Newman, SW: Manter and Gatz's Essentials of Clinical Neuroanatomy and Neurophysiology, ed 8. FA Davis, Philadelphia, 1992, p 49, with permission.)*

accidental emptying of the bladder will become more of a problem. The affected individual wets himself or herself because the bladder overflows after it fills to excess or it contracts reflexively before it is filled to capacity. Bladder pain, such as that which routinely occurs with urinary tract infections in women, is notably absent with the bladder problems caused by multiple sclerosis.

As with other symptoms of the demyelinating disease, the symptoms come and go unpredictably. With severe multiple sclerosis, the bladder problem may develop into a chronic disorder, but, in the early phases of the disease, it may be little more than a rare source of embarrassment. Techniques for minimizing bladder problems are discussed in Chapter 7.

Shifting Patterns of Symptoms

Regardless of what symptoms the individual develops, what suggests most that the problem is multiple sclerosis is a shifting pattern of complaints. A young person with bladder problems that come and go over the course of a few weeks who subsequently has depression and visual loss probably has multiple sclerosis. Regardless of what the initial signs of the disease are, about 65 percent of affected people will have complete resolution of the problem without any type of medical intervention. This complete resolution or remission will persist for days, months, or years, the duration of the remission being unrelated to the original sign or symptom. Even with recurrent symptoms for 5 or 6 years, the individual with multiple sclerosis may remain largely free of persistent or disabling nervous system problems.

Most neurologists believe that the diagnosis of multiple sclerosis should be reached only after the person has had two episodes that might reasonably be interpreted as attacks of demyelination. These injuries to the central nervous system should be separated by at least a month and should persist for at least 24 hours. The types of deficits should indicate that two different areas of the central nervous system have been involved.

Problems Found on Physical Examination (Signs)

What the physician finds on examining a person with multiple sclerosis may be dramatically different from what the person believes are the problems. Physical findings uncovered on examination are called the *signs,* rather than the symptoms, of the disease. Many obvious signs may go undetected by the person impaired by nervous system damage. Changes in speech, such as altered rhythms, are often unnoticed by the affected individual even after they are pointed out by the physician. Impaired sensation or clumsiness may be apparent only with specific tests. Some of the more common neurologic signs found on examining people with multiple sclerosis involve changes or deficits in eye movements, limb coordination, speech, and reflexes (Table 4–4).

Eye Signs

Aside from changes in visual acuity (the ability to see clearly), many other signs of multiple sclerosis involve the eyes. These include changes in the appearance of the optic nerve, abnormali-

---

TABLE 4–4. Common Signs of Multiple Sclerosis

Altered eye movements
Abnormal responses of the pupils
Paleness of the optic disc
Visual field disturbances
Overactive tendon reflexes
Limb spasticity
Localized weakness
Abnormal speech patterns
Circumscribed sensory disturbances

---

ties in eye movements or reflexes, and limitations in the field of vision (Table 4–5). Changes in the appearance of the optic disc, the point at which the optic nerve leaves the back of the eye, can be detected only with special equipment, but changes in eye movements, reflexes in response to light, and fields of vision can be checked with little more than a brightly colored pinhead and a flashlight.

A physician can examine the optic nerve by looking into the eye with a set of lenses called an *ophthalmoscope*. This type of examination may reveal atrophy (that is, degeneration) of the optic nerve. **Optic atrophy** is usually seen in people who have had obvious attacks of optic neuritis, inflammation in the optic nerve. The nerve looks paler than usual and the pattern of blood vessels on the nerve is slightly altered. Other changes in the eyes require little expertise to detect. Changes in the visual field are usually experienced as problems with visual acuity.

Light Reflex Changes

With damage to the optic nerve, the affected person has changes in the response of the pupils to light. The pupils are the black openings in the eyes through which light enters. The size of the pupil is determined by the colored ring of muscles that surrounds it, called *the iris*. The pupils normally constrict (or contract) in bright light because the iris narrows this opening and reduces the amount of light entering the eye. When a bright light is directed at either eye, both pupils become smaller as part of the consensual

---

TABLE 4–5. Common Eye Findings

Nystagmus
Optic nerve atrophy
Marcus Gunn pupil
Internuclear ophthalmoplegia
Impaired visual acuity
Centrocecal scotomas
Impaired color vision

(that is, normal) reflex response to the light, and the amount of change in both pupils is equal.

After optic neuritis, the affected eye has a less dramatic response to bright light than the unaffected eye, but still retains the consensual reflex. This produces the *Marcus Gunn pupil*—the curious pattern of a pupil constricting in the injured eye when a bright light is first shined into the good eye (consensual reflex) and then becoming somewhat larger (dilating) when the light is shined into the eye with optic atrophy (Figure 4–4). The pupil in the eye with optic atrophy dilates when the light is shined into it because this eye is less stimulated by direct light than it is by light

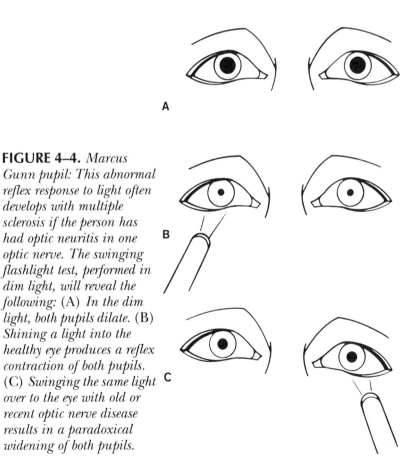

A

B

C

FIGURE 4–4. *Marcus Gunn pupil: This abnormal reflex response to light often develops with multiple sclerosis if the person has had optic neuritis in one optic nerve. The swinging flashlight test, performed in dim light, will reveal the following: (A) In the dim light, both pupils dilate. (B) Shining a light into the healthy eye produces a reflex contraction of both pupils. (C) Swinging the same light over to the eye with old or recent optic nerve disease results in a paradoxical widening of both pupils.*

that is perceived by the good eye. This Marcus Gunn pupil response may be the only sign of eye involvement in people with mild cases of multiple sclerosis. It is even seen when the individual cannot recall ever having had an episode of impaired vision.

Disturbed Eye Movements

Eye movements may be affected in a variety of ways. Large or small side-to-side or up-and-down movements, called **nystagmus,** may develop when the affected person looks to the sides or vertically. These are involuntary and may assume many different patterns. Specific patterns of nystagmus strongly suggest multiple sclerosis when they are found in young adults with other symptoms of scattered nervous system disease. One especially typical pattern occurs with **internuclear ophthalmoplegia.** With this disturbance of coordinated eye movements, nystagmus develops in the eye directed inward when looking to the side but does not appear when the eye turns inward to focus on an approaching object.

Reflex Changes

Reflexes in parts of the body other than the eyes may be altered with multiple sclerosis and yet produce no symptoms. The limbs have reflexes that can be seen by tapping with a small hammer on the tendons that connect muscles to bones. Normally, stretch receptors in the tendons perceive the abrupt change in the length of the tendon and convey this change along a sensory nerve fiber to the spinal cord. In the spinal cord, this information automatically activates nerve cells, or **neurons,** that directly or only slightly indirectly control the contraction of the muscle to which the stretched tendon is attached. Centers in the cerebellum and other parts of the brain and spinal cord adjust the forcefulness and persistence of the reflex contraction that occurs when these nerve cells are activated. All these interactions occur in a split second and ordinarily play a vital role in maintaining normal posture and accurate muscle activity.

If there has been subtle damage to the pathways in the brain or the spinal cord that modify the stretch reflex, there may be an obvious asymmetry in the strength of the observed tendon jerks. With damage to the motor pathways in the brain or in the spinal cord, these reflex tendon jerks are usually increased. If nerves to or from the muscles and tendons are damaged, the reflex may be entirely eliminated. With demyelinating disease, connections to and from the spinal cord are intact, but damage to the central nervous system pathways may result in greatly exaggerated sensitivity to stretching of the tendon. Sensitivity may be so exaggerated that stretching the tendon once causes repeated contractions in the attached muscle. This abnormal response is called **clonus** and is usually most easily seen at the ankle.

There are other reflexes involving distinct muscle responses that physicians often use to look for central nervous system disease. These include the Babinski reflex. Scraping the outside of the bottom of the foot normally causes the toes to curl downward, unless the individual is an infant (Figure 4–5). With damage to central nervous system motor pathways, the big toe will extend upward. This abnormal reflex response is called a positive *Babinski sign*. Other types of reflexes to touch and pain include retraction of a testicle when the adjacent thigh is scratched and contraction of the abdominal wall when part of the overlying skin is scratched. Disturbances of any of these reflexes suggest nervous system disease, but do not definitely establish the presence of demyelinating disease.

Weakness

Many of the pathways in the nervous system regulate strength and coordination. This means that damage in any one of a number of locations in the brain or spinal cord can produce problems with strength or with coordination of limb movements (see Figure 1–3). Problems with coordination may appear as problems with strength because the expression of full strength is limited by poor coordination of the muscles. For a movement to be executed with the intended force, both the contracting muscle and its opposing one must be acted on by the nervous system. The muscle responsi-

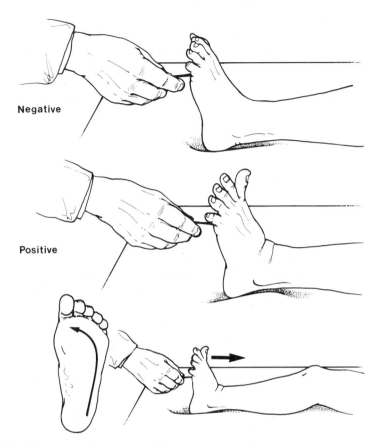

FIGURE 4–5. *Babinski sign: This abnormal reflex response to pain along the outside of the sole involves flaring of the small toes and upward movement of the big toe. (This response is not abnormal in infants.)*

ble for the movement must shorten and the opposing one must relax.

What is most distinctive in the weakness developing with multiple sclerosis is that it conforms to patterns typical of damage to the brain or spinal cord. Muscles supplied by more than one nerve are involved. The type of weakness occurring when a nerve in an arm or leg is cut or crushed is quite different. With such nerve injuries, a single muscle may be affected and problems with sensation usually appear over the area of skin supplied by the nerve. With injuries outside the central nervous system, **tone** (that is, the normal tension) in the affected muscles is decreased. With passive manipulation of the affected limb, little or no resistance occurs.

How the weakness developing with multiple sclerosis will manifest itself is unpredictable. It may appear as an inability to lift heavy weights, as a progressive loss of the ability to walk smoothly, or as easy fatigability. If a nerve in a limb is cut or crushed, the muscles it supplies lose both their normal tone and their normal mass or size. After a few weeks or months, little muscle tissue may be left. This is not true if the injury is in the central nervous system pathways that regulate strength and coordination. With damage to these pathways, tone increases and muscle mass diminishes only to the extent that the muscles are not used. This loss of bulk is called **disuse atrophy.** With severe weakness, it is unavoidable. The person loses muscle tissue simply because the muscle does not receive instructions to be active.

The degree of weakness that develops is not related to the individual's original level of strength. A weight lifter is no less likely to develop crippling weakness than a sedentary office worker. It is not the muscle itself that is impaired. It is the nervous system connections with the nerve cells that actually compel the muscle to be active. Indeed, it is not even the final nerve cell in the long chain of nerve cells that coordinates muscle activity that is disturbed. What is disturbed by demyelination is the system of nerve fibers above the last nerve cells in the system.

The outlook with weakness is quite unpredictable. No medical or surgical regimen has shown any promise in restoring strength that has been lost for months or years. Physical therapy will maximize the usefulness of the strength that remains, and the value of this cannot be overstated. Several types of physical therapy are discussed in Chapter 10.

Muscle Stiffness and Spasticity

Muscle tone, the tension in the muscle, is one of the most dramatically altered nervous system functions in many people with demyelinating disease. In most cases, it is increased if it is affected at all, and the increase in tone may be so extreme that it interferes with all useful movement of the affected limb. If the increase in tone depends on the rate at which the limb is moved, but the apparent resistance to movement is constant if the force applied across the joint is constant, the altered muscle tone is called *spasticity.* In other words, with spasticity, the resistance is greater the more rapidly the limb is moved. Relaxation of opposing muscles is inappropriately delayed even with passive manipulation of the limb (that is, movement by another person). Attempts to overcome spasticity by stretching the limbs or passively manipulating them may produce a great deal of pain.

Spasticity is a problem for the affected person because it interferes with normal movement of the limb even if strength is good or nearly intact. It may also cause substantial pain if limb strength is too poor to overcome the disabling positions into which the spasticity forces the limb. Spasticity may be so powerful that the contraction of the limb cannot be overcome even when a therapist tries to move the limb passively.

Whether the spasticity forces the affected arm or leg into a straight or bent position depends on the site of injury in the nervous system. The arm is almost always bent with severe spasticity, but the legs may be either bent or rigidly extended straight out. Obviously, a stiffly extended leg is easier to use than a stiffly flexed (bent) leg, but in either case the spasticity may be only part of the impairment in the limb. People with multiple sclerosis who have problems with walking often have a combination of weakness and spasticity in one or both legs, which produces a typical change in the way they walk. Because the leg is stiffly extended and strength in the leg is inadequate to bend the knee, the affected person may be obliged to swing the leg from the hip in a labored pattern, commonly referred to as **circumduction** (Figure 4–6).

When spasticity has forced a limb into a particular position for years, changes in the joints and the tendons around the affected joints may interfere with efforts to correct the position of the limb. Tendons may shorten and joints may freeze to the point that the position of the affected limb cannot be corrected even if all of the

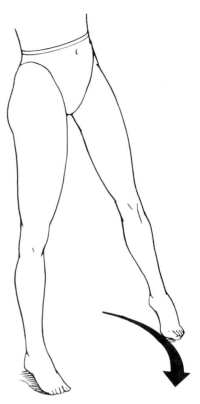

FIGURE 4–6. *Circumducting gait: With spasticity in one leg, the affected person may swing the impaired leg in a wide arc at the hip.*

original spasticity is eliminated. The limitations imposed by the spasticity become self-perpetuating.

Fortunately, these types of problems develop only with severe, prolonged spasticity. For most individuals with spasticity, clumsiness in the limb imposed by the abnormal tone is more disabling than the position the limb tends to assume. Unfortunately, spasticity rarely improves spontaneously. It most often develops to a significant degree in people who have an extensive or chronic progressive multiple sclerosis. A person who has had one or two minor flare-ups of demyelinating disease is much less likely to have any spasticity than one who has had recurrent, prolonged bouts of weakness. The person who does not fully recover strength after a flare-up is most likely to face the additional burden of spasticity. Physical therapy helps most if it is begun before spasticity has become severe, thereby maintaining as much normal muscle tone and motion as possible.

Although spontaneous remission is not characteristic of spasticity, there are several approaches to reducing or eliminating it, including therapy, medication, and surgery. These are discussed in Chapter 7.

Sensory Disturbances

A complete loss of sensation over a limited area of the body may go completely unnoticed by the affected person until a systematic examination of pain and touch perception reveals it. With loss of pain perception in the fingers, the individual may develop burns or ulcers during smoking, cooking, or other routine activities. This type of anesthesia (that is, loss of all sensation) sometimes does occur with extreme cases of multiple sclerosis, but, in most cases, the sensory disturbance caused by MS is slightly impaired

TABLE 4–6. Pain

Causes	*Common Sites*
Infection	Bladder (cystitis)
	Skin (cellulitis)
	Bone (osteomyelitis)
Contusion	Tendons
	Ligaments
Dislocation	Shoulder
	Hip
Fracture	Wrist
	Ribs
	Ankle
	Spine
Sensory pathway injury	Face
	Limbs
	Trunk

perception of pain, touch, or temperature, often associated with recurrent attacks of pain over limited areas (focal deficits).

If pain develops in a fairly circumscribed area, the affected person must be investigated for local problems, such as infections or fractures (Table 4–6). Pain in the knee may be from contusion (bruising) of a knee ligament. Pain in the back or neck may be from a spinal fracture. Pain over the trunk may be from a local infection. Deciding whether any pain is from damage to nervous system pathways or a local injury requires the expertise of a physician.

One type of unusual pain that may be found by a physician considering the diagnosis of multiple sclerosis is that experienced when the neck is bent forward rapidly. With central nervous system demyelination, this maneuver may cause an electric sensation radiating down the spine (Figure 4–7). This is called **Lhermitte's sign,** and it may be found on examination of people with multiple sclerosis who have no other signs of sensory damage.

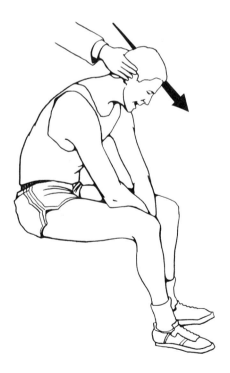

FIGURE 4–7. *Lhermitte's sign: Briskly flexing the neck forward may produce an electric sensation running down the spine or into the limbs in people with multiple sclerosis.*

Why this abnormal sensation occurs with multiple sclerosis is unknown even though it has been recognized for decades. It occurs in other nervous system diseases, but it suggests multiple sclerosis when it appears with other typical signs, such as bladder disturbances or visual problems.

The sensory problems developing with multiple sclerosis are usually short-lived and inconsistent. A notable exception is the facial pain of trigeminal neuralgia. Years after all other signs of multiple sclerosis have stabilized or disappeared, the severe, sudden pains that are so typical of and disabling in trigeminal neuralgia may persist. Fortunately, this complication of the central nervous system disease can be treated (see Chapter 7).

Significance of Signs and Symptoms

These signs and symptoms of disease can be properly interpreted only by an experienced physician. Individuals should not try to decide whether or not they have multiple sclerosis on the basis of their own perception of their signs and symptoms. Even the patient's own symptoms require an objective interviewer to allow a complete picture to emerge. An experienced physician can weigh the significance of various symptoms and determine if they are related to any physical findings. If the entire picture suggests that multiple sclerosis is the cause of the individual's problems, further diagnostic tests, as discussed in Chapter 5, may be used to increase the certainty of the diagnosis.

Diagnostic Tests

N o blood test, X-ray study, or other type of objective examination will establish without doubt that a person's complaints arise from multiple sclerosis, but there are many techniques that help the physician reach the diagnosis with considerable confidence (Table 5–1). The structural changes in the brain and the spinal cord that are typical or multiple sclerosis are still not easily seen with X ray and other imaging techniques, but that is changing. Some of the more recently developed equipment, such as magnetic resonance imaging (MRI) machines, will reveal some plaques, but other types of damage to the nervous system can be mistaken for plaques. Although no single test is highly reliable, findings consistent with multiple sclerosis on several tests and signs or symptoms typical of the disease on clinical evaluation of the patient allow an unequivocal decision in most cases.

Spinal Fluid Examination

The entire brain and spinal cord is bathed in a clear, colorless fluid called *cerebrospinal fluid* or, more simply, spinal fluid. This fluid circulates around the brain and the spinal cord, providing a

TABLE 5–1. Diagnostic Tests

Test	Finding
Cerebrospinal fluid	Usually abnormal protein composition
Visual evoked potentials	Latency prolonged (same changes with all causes of optic neuritis, optic nerve compression, and other causes of visual loss)
Computed tomography (CT) of the brain	Scattered areas of increased density (white patches on high-contrast CT)
Magnetic resonance imaging (MRI)	Scattered areas of abnormal nerve tissue

shock-absorbing environment for the entire central nervous system. Specific elements in the central nervous system constantly produce and reabsorb this fluid and maintain its pressure and composition. Ordinarily, it is almost completely free of cells and has very little protein. The few cells that normally are found in the fluid are white blood cells with simple internal features. The proteins normally in the fluid are varied and complex, but as long as the individual is healthy, the variety and concentration of proteins are fairly constant.

Changes in the nervous system caused by many diseases affect the composition of this fluid. Multiple sclerosis is one of the diseases that produce characteristic changes in the cerebrospinal fluid (Table 5–2), but none of the changes developing with multiple sclerosis is unique. All the abnormalities induced by multiple sclerosis may occur with some infections, with other demyelinating diseases, and with central nervous system diseases of unknown cause. With multiple sclerosis, proteins associated with the myelin of the central nervous system, called *myelin basic proteins,* are often found in higher-than-normal concentrations. These myelin basic proteins are a crude measure of the extent of myelin damage in the central nervous system, and they are also higher than normal with other diseases that cause substantial myelin damage.

Some of the proteins associated with immune reactions, called

TABLE 5–2. Cerebrospinal Fluid in Multiple Sclerosis

Pressure	Normal
Appearance	Normal
Cell count	Normal or slightly increased white blood cells
Protein content	Normal or slightly elevated
Gamma globulin	More than 15% of total protein
Oligoclonal bands	Positive in 85%–90% with MS False positive in 4% of all patients IgG typically increased

antibodies or **immunoglobulins,** also appear in abnormal patterns. The biochemical techniques used for identifying these antibodies or immunoglobulins in the cerebrospinal fluid display the various classes of immunoglobulin proteins as bands on paper or in gelatin columns. With multiple sclerosis, there may be a characteristic increase in **gamma globulin,** one of the immunoglobulins important in the response of the immune system to disease. Only a few of the many possible immunoglobulins in the fluid are increased by the disease to a sufficient concentration to appear as unusually distinct bands on the paper or gel used to separate them. This is called **oligoclonal banding,** a term that literally means there are excessive amounts of a few families of immunoglobulin proteins. If an individual has evidence of demyelinating disease in the central nervous system and has this typical pattern of immunoglobulin proteins in the cerebrospinal fluid, the likelihood that the cause of the disease is multiple sclerosis is about 85 percent.

The class of immunoglobulin proteins or antibodies that is usually elevated in the cerebrospinal fluid of patients with multiple sclerosis is the immunoglobulin G (IgG) group. These proteins are antibodies to unknown substances. This IgG protein is assembled from other protein constituents that can be examined individually. Current investigations of these antibodies indicate that people with multiple sclerosis have a component protein chain, called the *light chain,* that has a typical composition, called *kappa.* An elevated kappa-chain content of the cerebrospinal fluid may be a better indicator of multiple sclerosis than the finding of increased levels of IgG alone, but even this biochemical finding is not proof that the person has multiple sclerosis.

To get cerebrospinal fluid, the physician must stick a needle into the space in which the fluid circulates. This is usually done below the spinal cord at the base of the spine and is called a *lumbar puncture* or *spinal tap.* Many people are concerned about having a spinal tap, but the concern is not warranted if the procedure is performed by an experienced physician.

The space in which cerebrospinal fluid circulates over the brain and about the spinal cord is called the *subarachnoid space.* This space is formed by the tough wrappings that surround the central nervous system, and it extends several inches below the end of the spinal cord.

Fluid obtained by sticking a needle into the subarachnoid space in this region or elsewhere is replaced within a few hours. After the sample of fluid is removed for testing, the person with multiple sclerosis should have no new complaints. Many people do complain of a headache, but this usually lasts only a few hours if it develops at all. The headache is believed to result from a reduction in the volume or pressure of the cerebrospinal fluid. Limiting the person's activity and keeping him or her flat in bed for a few hours after the spinal tap is usually sufficient to minimize the headache. Even when a severe headache develops, it does not indicate any new problems in the nervous system. Taking pain killers, drinking lots of fluids, and restricting activity are the only appropriate measures for managing the headache once it appears.

Evoked Potential and Other Electrical Studies

Electrical studies of the brain have been available for decades, but over the past 15 years special techniques have been developed for more accurately studying the transmission of information in relatively small areas of the brain. Electrical activity in the brain reaches the surface of the skin and can be monitored by attaching fine wires to the scalp with glue or pins. Signals picked up by these wires must be greatly amplified with specially designed equipment before they can be examined.

Electroencephalography

Electrical activity in the outer layers of the brain can be monitored with an amplifying device called an **electroencephalograph (EEG).** Although this electrical activity is called *brain-wave activity,* it is a reliable indicator of activity only in the most superficial layers of the brain. This activity may also be abnormal with damage to deeper brain structures, but it is less reliable as a test of disturbed brain pathways, such as those likely to be injured with multiple sclerosis. Therefore, an EEG study of a person with extensive demyelination from multiple sclerosis may show normal brain waves.

    Electroencephalography is routinely performed on individuals believed to have multiple sclerosis, because this technique may suggest another basis for the signs and symptoms. Some of the infectious diseases that cause neurologic problems similar to multiple sclerosis will produce characteristic changes in the brain waves detected by the EEG machine. Changes suggestive of epilepsy would also point away from the diagnosis of MS since epilepsy is not a neurologic complication of multiple sclerosis.

Evoked Potential Studies

By giving a person specific stimuli, such as flashing lights, clicking noises, shifting checkerboard patterns, and electrical shocks, physicians can evoke (elicit) reproducible patterns of electrical activity in the central nervous system. These patterns of electrical activity caused by specific stimuli are called **evoked potentials.** Each type of evoked potential consists of a series of waves (Figure 5–1). Each of these waves reflects electrical activity in a limited part of the nervous system. As the signal elicited by the stimulus is

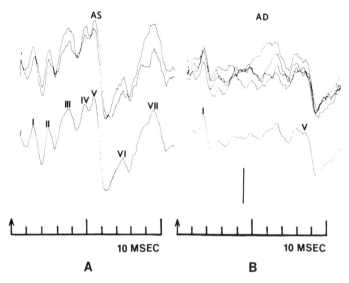

FIGURE 5–1. *Brain-stem auditory evoked potential. The patient's left ear (A) is normal. The patient has an affected right ear (B). The changes in the spacing or the shape of the brain waves evoked by repeated stimuli may reveal unexpected brain-stem disease in the person with multiple sclerosis. (From Poser, CM et al: The Diagnosis of Multiple Sclerosis. Thieme Medical Publishers, New York, 1984, p 121, with permission.)*

transported along nerve pathways, it activates centers that process, redistribute, or amplify the information. Major centers of activity produce characteristic waves in the split second after the the stimulus that is monitored by the evoked potential equipment.

A clicking noise will produce an auditory or **brain-stem auditory evoked potential** (see Figure 5–1). A shifting checkerboard pattern on a screen directly in front of the individual will elicit a **visual evoked potential**. Electrical shocks to the arms or legs or over the spine will produce **somatosensory evoked potentials.**

Changes in any of these evoked potentials is not strong evidence of multiple sclerosis or even of demyelinating disease. Other types of nervous system disease ranging from tumors to infections can disturb the evoked potentials. What makes these studies useful is that they may uncover an unsuspected problem in part of the nervous system not directly related to where the individual initially had complaints. The person with bladder problems may prove to have an abnormal visual evoked potential. This would make multiple sclerosis a more likely explanation for the bladder problem.

This type of study carries no risks. The equipment used merely records normal activity that is generated by the brain and spinal cord in response to a harmless stimulus. It is, however, relatively expensive and will be replaced by more informative tests, such as magnetic resonance imaging, when the costs of these even more expensive tests decline.

Computed Tomography of the Brain

Computed tomography of the brain (CT scan) is an imaging technique that uses X rays to construct a picture of the brain. A computer analyzes the absorption of X rays by brain structures of differing densities to create the image (Figure 5–2). The density

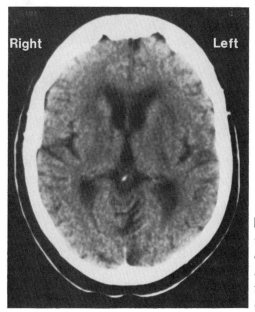

FIGURE 5–2. *The CT scan uses X rays to measure the density of structures in the head and usually does not reveal areas of demyelination. This is a normal scan.*

of blood and bone are very different from that of the brain, so a variety of structures, both normal and abnormal, can be readily identified with this technique. Injecting a person with a fluid, called *contrast material,* that circulates through the blood vessels in the head and that is relatively opaque to X rays helps to show structures with many blood vessels. Computed tomography has provided considerable insight into the structure of the brain in a number of diseases, but its usefulness with multiple sclerosis is limited.

In multiple sclerosis, the changes in the brain occurring with a flare-up may involve very little tissue. The smallest volume of tissue well visualized by most CT equipment is a few cubic millimeters, but a major neurologic problem may occur with lesions much smaller than this. Even large plaques of demyelination may be difficult to see because the density of the plaque is not strikingly different from that of normal tissue. Some plaques can be seen after injection of large doses of the contrast material because the character of the blood vessels in the plaque may be different enough (white) from that in surrounding tissues to enhance the contrast perceived by the machine (Figure 5–3).

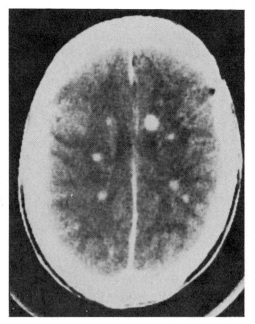

FIGURE 5–3. *CT scan with flare-up of MS: With high-dose contrast material, plaques of demyelination may be seen as white patches on the CT scan. (From Poser, CM et al: The Diagnosis of Multiple Sclerosis. Thieme Medical Publishers, New York, 1984, p 198, with permission.)*

Even when areas of abnormal tissue are revealed by the computed tomogram, they cannot be identified confidently as demyelinated plaques. Tumors, infections, and small strokes may look very much like damage from demyelination. Much of the damage caused by multiple sclerosis is in the spinal cord, and this part of the central nervous system is especially difficult to visualize with computed tomography. The spinal cord is only millimeters thick along much of its length, so a change in the cord that can cause considerable paralysis is usually imperceptible with computed tomography.

Except for the contrast material injection, this procedure is entirely risk-free and painless. The contrast material occasionally causes allergic reactions in people sensitive to iodine, but the facilities that use this technique generally are prepared to manage an allergic reaction. Because this approach usually does not help in identifying demyelination in the brain, its principal value is in ruling out other structural lesions in the brain. It is widely available but is still relatively expensive.

Magnetic Resonance Imaging

Magnetic resonance imaging (MRI) or nuclear magnetic resonance (NMR) is one of the newest diagnostic techniques available to neurologists, and it has provided considerable assistance in the investigation of multiple sclerosis. It uses magnetic waves to analyze the composition of tissues. The system, which analyzes changes in tissue responses to a shifting magnetic field, is similar to that used in computed tomography. Plaques of demyelination are likely to appear with high resolution with this technique (Figure 5–4). Determining that an area of damage is actually demyelination rather than a tumor or an injury involving a blood vessel is somewhat simpler with magnetic resonance imaging than with computed tomography because the magnetic technique reveals many of the plaques not evident with computed tomography. The appearance of numerous areas of injury scattered throughout the nervous system, including some in the spinal cord, strongly suggests multiple sclerosis (Figure 5–5).

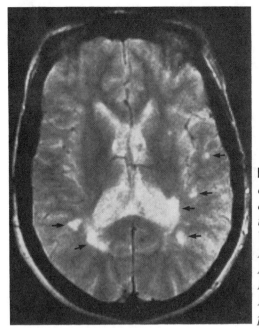

FIGURE 5–4. *The plaques of multiple sclerosis show up as white patches (arrows) on this MRI scan. (From Wolpert, S: Neuroimaging. In Bradley, WG et al [eds]: Neurology in Clinical Practice. Butterworth-Heinemann, Boston, 1991, p 523, with permission.)*

Individuals with metal implants, such as cardiac pacemakers, cannot tolerate the magnetic field generated for the MRI study. Otherwise, there is no reason why a person cannot have this scan. The study is painless and appears to be risk-free. Some physicians are injecting materials into the people they study to increase the information provided by the imaging technique. People who are allergic to such material may have adverse reactions, but these are usually limited to rashes and fevers that disappear within hours. The technique is still not readily available in some places and is very expensive.

Myelography

Whenever an individual develops signs of a spinal cord injury, the physician must determine the best way to investigate the problem. The most sensitive technique currently available for evaluating

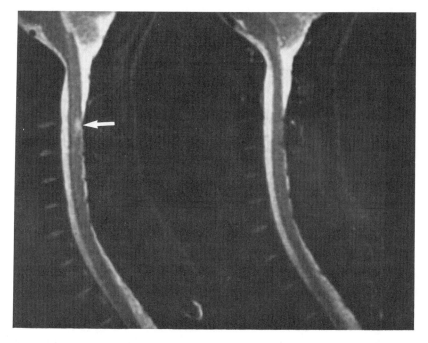

FIGURE 5–5. *MRI shows an MS plaque (arrow) in the spinal cord of this 27-year-old woman. The fact that the spinal cord is not enlarged particularly suggests that this area is a plaque rather than a tumor or other type of lesion. (From Drayer, BP: Magnetic Resonance Imaging of Adult White Matter Disease. In Mazziotta, JC and Gilman, S [eds]: Clinical Brain Imaging: Principles and Applications. FA Davis, Philadelphia, 1992, p 359, with permission.)*

spinal cord damage is myelography. With this technique, a relatively opaque dye is put into the cerebrospinal fluid, usually by way of a lumbar puncture. The person is tilted on a board as X-ray pictures are taken of the spine with the dye outlining the spinal cord. The dye flows in the space around the spinal cord and reveals irregularities or obstructions. A tumor pressing on the spinal cord or a cyst originating in the spinal cord will be easily revealed with this technique.

Demyelinating plaques produce no changes that are visible on a myelogram (the X ray), but myelography is occasionally done on people with multiple sclerosis before the diagnosis is evident. If an individual's first complaint is loss of bowel and bladder control with weakness in both legs, myelography will usually be performed on an emergency basis. If multiple sclerosis is the cause of the problem, nothing is lost by doing the study.

Myelography is done as an emergency because the chances of reversing damage caused by spinal cord compression decrease rapidly if the pressure on the cord is allowed to continue for days. The problems occurring with multiple sclerosis are usually temporary, so the affected individual does not suffer permanent harm if the investigation is delayed, but most people considered for myelography do not yet have the diagnosis of multiple sclerosis established for them. The person who develops weakness and numbness in both legs after prior episodes of visual loss, slurred speech, clumsiness, and bladder problems will rarely be investigated with myelography.

Myelography is a relatively safe, but fairly uncomfortable, procedure. In addition to having a spinal tap, the patient must lie face down on a hard surface for several minutes to an hour while the study is performed. Most people complain of headache after myelography, and a few are allergic to the material injected. The procedure must be performed in a hospital but may not require more than one day of confinement.

Treatment of Multiple Sclerosis

There is no cure for multiple sclerosis, but there are many types of treatment for managing acute exacerbations and complications of the disease. For some individuals with multiple sclerosis, management of the flare-ups is the most significant part of treatment because few or no chronic problems remain after the flare-up resolves. Unfortunately, this is a relatively small fraction of all people with MS. With the introduction of interferon beta-1b (Betaseron), an agent that appears to reduce the frequency of exacerbations in some individuals with relapsing-remitting MS is available.

About 20 percent of those who have had multiple sclerosis diagnosed on the basis of typical signs or symptoms have only minor disabilities after 20 years of disease regardless of what type of treatment they receive. The severity of complications for the remaining 80 percent of the population is extraordinarily diverse and unpredictable. Management of the chronic problems that may develop with multiple sclerosis is discussed in Chapter 7.

Complicating the assessment of any therapy is a phenomenon called the *placebo effect*. A *placebo* is a drug or other substance that is known to be ineffective against a medical problem, such as multiple sclerosis. For a medical study to establish that a treatment

79

works against multiple sclerosis, the substance being tested must be compared with a placebo. Some people in the medical study are given the placebo but are not told they are receiving an ineffective substance. Nevertheless, their belief that the substance might work will often produce a positive result (the placebo effect), which is especially likely to complicate the interpretation of a medical study involving a disease with an unpredictable course. If the substance being tested produces a better outcome than the placebo, the researchers may conclude that it is useful in treating the disease.

New Therapy with Interferon

Interferon is a protein normally produced by the body. It was first recognized because of its ability to interfere with viral infection. There are at least three different types of interferons: alpha, beta, and gamma. Each type of interferon has a distinct chemical composition and exerts a wide range of effects over the immune and other systems in the body. Because these proteins affect the functioning of the immune system, they were tried in the treatment of individuals with multiple sclerosis. Early studies using gamma interferon suggested that this protein worsened the problems faced by the patient with relapsing-remitting MS. In comparison with a placebo, at least one form of beta interferon, interferon beta-1b (Betaseron), has had a beneficial effect in individuals with relapsing-remitting MS who are able to walk. The only people with multiple sclerosis studied in this kind of large, placebo-controlled clinical trial of interferon beta-1b have all had relatively mild disease. Studies of another beta interferon (interferon beta-1a) have revealed similar benefits in individuals with MS given this material for 2 years.

Interferon Beta-1b

Interferon beta-1b differs slightly from naturally occurring human beta interferon and is produced by genetically altered bacteria (*Escherichia coli* or *E. coli*), rather than by being taken directly from any animals. Studies in people with multiple sclerosis using interferon beta-1b compared two doses—1.6 million international units (mIU) and 8 mIU—of this drug to a placebo. (The international units used refer to inhibition of viral activity and have nothing to do with multiple sclerosis.) The test substances (interferon or a placebo) were injected just under the skin (subcutaneously) every other day. After 2 years of treatment, the groups getting interferon beta-1b had significantly fewer flare-ups than the group getting placebo. The number of days during which subjects had moderate or severe exacerbations was, on average, less for the high-dose group than for the placebo group.

Magnetic resonance imaging (MRI) was used to examine the people in this study (see Chapter 5). The scans of the brains of those who received the higher dose of interferon beta-1b showed less of the type of activity generally considered undesirable than the scans of people who received a placebo. Precisely what was less active in the brain—demyelination, inflammation, or some other process—is not known for sure, but MRI does appear to be a useful method for evaluating the effectiveness of proposed treatments. The results shown by those receiving interferon beta-1b are especially encouraging because a similar study of cyclosporine, a drug that interferes with the immune system, did not produce this kind of result on MRI.

Most individuals getting either the high dose or the low dose of interferon beta-1b experienced some side effects. The most common were skin reactions at the injection sites, flu-like symptoms, pain, and short-term weakness or fatigue. These flu-like symptoms consisted of fever, chills, muscle aches, headache, and joint pains. At the injection sites, many people developed reddening, hardening, and sensitivity of the skin similar to that associated with an insect bite. The most worrisome side effects were changes in blood tests that suggest abnormal liver function, as well as disturbances of mood, such as emotional lability, depression, and suicidal thoughts. Many individuals had a decrease in their white blood cell counts and some women had menstrual irregularities. After considering the apparent benefits and risks of interferon beta-1b therapy, the Food and Drug Administration (FDA) approved it "for use in ambulatory patients with relapsing-remitting multiple sclerosis to reduce the frequency of clinical exacerbations.''

The recommended dose of interferon beta-1b is 8 mIU every other day. It is supplied as a freeze-dried powder to which a salt solution (diluent) must be added before it is injected under the skin. How long individuals should remain on this therapy to achieve maximum benefit is unknown.

Other Interferons

Tests of other beta interferons, administered by alternative methods on different schedules, are under way. Interferon beta-1a, for example, has been used in studies in people with multiple sclerosis on a once-weekly basis, given by injections into muscle. These studies are looking at whether or not the progression of disability is delayed in individuals getting this form of beta interferon and preliminary reports suggest that it probably does.

Studies using **alpha interferons** have been attempted by some investigators with varying success. Alpha interferon is structurally similar to beta interferon. Effects similar to those observed with beta interferon are thought to exist but have not yet been proven. The side effects with alpha interferon are as severe as, if not more severe than, those occurring with beta interferon and preliminary reports suggest that it probably does.

Long-Term Therapy

After the first episode of neurologic problems, most people with multiple sclerosis have a complete recovery. The earliest signs and symptoms of multiple sclerosis clear relatively quickly and completely regardless of how they are managed. This is part of the reason why many treatment approaches seem to work at first but subsequently produce no change in the course of the illness. To identify a therapy that truly affects the course of multiple sclerosis, physicians need to observe many individuals treated over several years.

Because the signs and symptoms of multiple sclerosis usually abate spontaneously after a flare-up, it is difficult to know if a drug used to suppress the disease worked or simply did not interfere with the normal course of the illness. With some diseases, the person's survival with and without treatment can be compared, but survival data are of no value in evaluating treatment of a disease like multiple sclerosis. Whether or not someone with MS survives longer with a treatment is not a reliable indicator of how effective the approach is, for multiple sclerosis is not a lethal problem. Its most severe complications, such as depression and urinary tract disturbances, may be life-threatening if they are not managed properly, but the central nervous system disorder itself is not fatal. What any effective long-term therapy must do is to improve the general condition of individuals treated over the course of years. Currently no treatment has been proven to substantially affect the long-term outlook.

What is not clear is whether or not therapies that reduce the severity or frequency of individual flare-ups of the disease will affect the status of the individual after 10 to 20 years of disease. Exacerbations of multiple sclerosis do respond to drug therapy, but most physicians are convinced that the problems seen months or years after the flare-up are probably not reduced or altered by treating the acute exacerbation. What is altered is the duration of the attack.

Of course, minimizing the severity of flare-ups and decreasing the frequency with which they occur are important. Many of the complications of multiple sclerosis develop because of the time out of each year spent with severe nervous system disturbances. Simply shortening the duration of a flare-up or decreasing the number of flare-ups each year may reduce the risk of complications. It will certainly decrease the stress faced during the flare-up and reduce the time each year spent in a hospital or at home managing the flare-up.

Therapy for Flare-Ups

There are many different approaches to the management of flare-ups. Some are well established. Most are controversial and will not survive protracted scrutiny. Regardless of what approach is used, the initiation of treatment for an exacerbation should be delayed for a few days or a week whenever that is feasible. This allows spontaneous improvements to become evident and spares the affected person unnecessary drug treatment or other procedures.

This delay is often foregone when the individual has severe multiple sclerosis with past episodes that routinely failed to improve quickly. The type of neurologic problem developing with the flare-up necessarily influences the decision of whether or not to delay treatment. If the affected person develops severe pain and complete loss of vision in one eye, few neurologists would delay treatment with corticosteroids or adrenocorticotropic hormone (**ACTH**) (see below). Even if the amount of vision retained is not affected by treatment, other considerations, such as alleviation of pain, will prompt the physician to start treatment as soon as the problem develops. On the other hand, the abrupt appearance of a pins-and-needles sensation in one hand or mild clumsiness in one foot does not justify early intervention with therapy that carries its own risks.

Individuals receiving beta interferon will still have flare-ups, but the flare-ups are generally less frequent than would be expected if they took a placebo or had no treatment. A flare-up has not been considered a basis for stopping treatment with beta interferon. Treatment with corticosteroids or ACTH has been used during flare-ups in people taking beta interferon. Whether this is appropriate or useful is still controversial.

Corticosteroids and ACTH

ACTH is the most widely used agent for managing acute flare-ups. This hormone is a substance produced by the brain. It is vital in the regulation of the adrenal glands, glands that sit on top of the kidneys and produce steroids, a variety of substances essential for life. Corticosteroids, one family of steroids, have been used to manage the signs and symptoms of flare-ups with some success, but the side effects of these drugs led physicians to look for equally effective alternatives. ACTH is one of the alternatives developed.

ACTH was first used in the management of multiple sclerosis because it yields the benefits of corticosteroid treatment with fewer of the side effects. The most troublesome complication of corticosteroid use is that it suppresses the adrenal glands' production of natural steroids. If the adrenal gland stops producing its own steroids for a period of weeks, life-threatening problems with blood pressure control, blood chemistry regulation, and other essential activities may develop when the prescribed drugs are stopped suddenly. Because ACTH does not stop the adrenal glands' work, these life-threatening problems do not occur.

A long-debated question surrounding the use of corticosteroids and ACTH has been whether their use in early treatment of multiple sclerosis has any effect on the course (outcome) of the disease. Because inflammation of the nerve from the eye (optic neuritis) is one of the most common problems early in the natural history of multiple sclerosis, many investigators have tried to monitor the course of people with optic neuritis who receive corticosteroids and later prove to have multiple sclerosis. Optic neuritis is often the first sign of multiple sclerosis, with other signs and symptoms developing in the following months or years. It is generally accepted that the long-term outcome after the early use of corticosteroids is similar to what would have happened if they had not been used at all. Whether or not there are short-term advantages to using corticosteroids, aside from the obvious ones of reducing discomfort and shortening the duration of flare-ups, has been more difficult to resolve.

Recent experience with corticosteroid treatment of optic neuritis suggests that there may be short-term advantages to using this type of therapy before full-blown multiple sclerosis develops. In individuals treated with intravenous (that is, injected into the vein) **methylprednisolone,** a corticosteroid often used to treat multiple sclerosis flare-ups, followed by oral prednisone (another corticosteroid), multiple sclerosis evolved at a lower rate over the next 2 years than in people with optic neuritis treated with oral prednisone alone or with a placebo.

Why this intravenous methylprednisolone made so obvious a

difference in the course of multiple sclerosis in people with optic neuritis is unknown. It is especially puzzling since the intravenous methylprednisolone was given for only 3 days, and the oral prednisone appears to be very well-absorbed into the bloodstream and just as active as the methylprednisolone once it is there. The importance of these observations is still unknown, but the observations are prompting a closer look at long-standing practices in the management of flare-ups.

Mechanisms of Action

Corticosteroids and ACTH are both of value in managing acute episodes of demyelination. Both drugs suppress the production of antibodies in the central nervous system. Whether this is the basis for their effect is not known. Whatever the mechanism by which they influence the flare-up, these drugs probably do not affect the total damage done during specific episodes, but they do shorten the duration of the episode.

Some investigators believe that ACTH influences the disease by altering concentrations of fluid in the central nervous system. During a flare-up, the tissues in the area of inflammation swell, and it is conceivable that by simply reducing the swelling, the nerve fibers in the region will work better. Corticosteroids and ACTH can both reduce some types of swelling, called *edema.* The importance of this effect is controversial.

As already mentioned, ACTH causes the adrenal glands to produce and release steroids, such as **cortisone,** that affect a wide variety of body systems. One of the most dramatic effects of steroid treatment is the reduction of inflammation which is the body's natural response to injury. Much of the activity observed in demyelination resembles natural responses to injury, so giving drugs that suppress the body's response to injury has long had its supporters. Many physicians believe that steroids are useful in reducing the time required for recovery from a flare-up. That steroids should be used rather than ACTH is controversial, but many physicians find them as effective as ACTH and much simpler to administer.

Corticosteroids, such as prednisone, cortisone acetate, and

dexamethasone, may be taken orally. They can be self-administered, and the dosage can be adjusted daily. Methylprednisolone is also widely used, but it is administered intravenously. Taking these drugs usually gives an individual a feeling of well-being. This may be misinterpreted as actual improvement in the disease, but even the illusion of improvement may be beneficial.

In some situations, such as in the treatment of optic neuritis, most physicians will use steroids for flare-ups of multiple sclerosis. When the optic nerve is painfully inflamed and vision deteriorates or ceases abruptly but no other neurologic signs appear, the physician may give steroids to reduce inflammation in the nerve and thereby reduce pain in the eye. ACTH is not as useful as steroids in the management of the pain. It is not clear whether vision can actually be helped by this maneuver, but management of the pain alone is a major consideration and justifies the use of the drugs.

Usual Dosages

The usual dose of ACTH administered in the treatment of flare-ups is 40 international units (IU) daily, given intravenously or injected into muscle, for 3 weeks. Most physicians reduce the total daily dose when 1 or 2 weeks have passed or when the individual shows substantial improvement. Although ACTH is not a steroid, it does promote the increased formation of steroids that, in turn, will lead to problems with blood pressure and blood sugar regulation over the course of weeks or months. Every person taking ACTH must be observed closely. In some people, hypertension (high blood pressure) or diabetes mellitus may develop, but these routinely abate when the drug is stopped.

Repeated cycles of ACTH therapy may be given with no apparent cumulative effects of the treatment over the course of a decade. Some individuals may need several cycles of treatment in a year. In either case, the problems caused by the exacerbations are not reduced except to the extent that prolonged disability during each flare-up produces its own problems.

Several types of corticosteroids are used widely. Cortisone can be taken as a tablet of cortisone acetate or as an intravenous solution, but more powerful corticosteroid preparations are preferred by most physicians who administer these drugs. Prednisone is often given at an initial oral dose of 80 to 200 milligrams (mg) daily for 1 week, followed by decreasing doses of the drug over the course of 2 weeks. Methylprednisolone, given intravenously, will shorten the duration of flare-ups in some people with multiple sclerosis, and, as discussed above, some physicians believe it can actually increase the likelihood of improvement. Dexamethasone (Decadron) is also widely used; the required dose is about one tenth that of prednisone.

The major side effects of steroid treatment include reversible changes in several different body systems. With long-term use, most people will develop rounding of the face and more obvious facial hair. Some will develop high blood pressure or diabetes mellitus after a relatively brief exposure to the medications, and so blood pressure and blood sugar levels must be monitored in any person started on these drugs. Prolonged treatment with high doses of the drugs will cause blood pressure and blood sugar problems in most people. Both of these problems will subside after the individual stops taking steroids. Resistance to infection is lowered, and thinning of bones is likely. Changes in the skeleton over the course of months may produce fractures.

ACTH with Cyclophosphamide

Because the impact of ACTH on the long-term course of multiple sclerosis is negligible, other drugs have been tried in combination with the hormone. The rationale for this combination is that ACTH alone clearly affects flare-ups, so with another drug helping it, ACTH may exert a more lasting effect. The drugs currently preferred in association with ACTH are medications that suppress the body's own immune system (Figure 6–1). These are called immunosuppresants (Table 6–1). The most promising results have been observed with cyclophosphamide (Cytoxan), but several other agents, such as azathioprine (Imuran), cyclosporine,

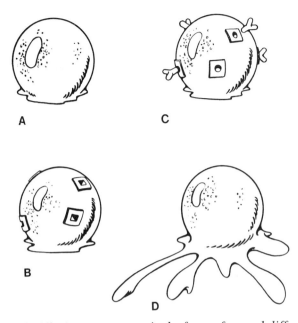

FIGURE 6–1. *The immune system is the focus of several different therapies. It consists of many cell types working together to fight off infection. White blood cells are especially important and include two different types of lymphocytes referred to as T cells (A) and B cells (B). (C) B cells develop into antibody-producing cells. (D) T cells interact with scavenger cells called macrophages.*

CCNU, 5-fluorocytosine, methotrexate, and cytarabine, are under investigation or have been used in studies of people with MS.

Experience with ACTH and cyclophosphamide in combination has been relatively limited, but some studies have been promising. A few have shown a slight, but significant, tendency for combined therapy to reduce the number and severity of flare-ups of multiple sclerosis. Some investigators claim that they have seen stabilization of progressive multiple sclerosis for 1 to 3 years in 75 percent of individuals treated for 10 to 14 days with combined intravenous cyclophosphamide and ACTH. The results ascribed to the cyclophosphamide have been observed after relatively short trials of the drug. This makes the results more promising, because there are still many dosage schedules that can be tried.

TABLE 6–1. Drugs Used to Suppress Immunity

Hormones
ACTH
Steroids
Cortisone acetate
Prednisone
Methylprednisolone
Dexamethasone
Other Immunosuppressant Drugs
Cyclophosphamide
Azathioprine
CCNU
5-Fluorocytosine
Cytarabine
Methotrexate
Cop-1

The major disadvantage of cyclophosphamide is that it affects the blood and other tissues adversely when used in high doses. It may supress blood production by the bone marrow or irritate the lining of the bladder. This immunosuppressant (that is, an agent that inhibits the immune system) has been used for other diseases, such as leukemia and cancer, for several years, so the long-term consequences of exposure to the drug are better known than are the consequences of exposure to other treatments that are currently being tried. Although experience with the drug is extensive, the full extent of complications likely to be experienced by an individual with multiple sclerosis cannot be known until several thousand people with the disease have been exposed to the immunosuppressant.

The complications of cyclophosphamide that are known are disturbing. Early after treatment with the drug, considerable hair loss and bleeding disorders (often affecting the bladder) occur routinely. The bone marrow is sensitive to this drug, and so blood reactions must be watched for during the first few weeks after exposure to the drug. This is certainly not a harmless treatment, but if it truly affects the frequency and severity of flare-ups, it will be worth the risk.

From all experience, it is clear that cyclophosphamide is a potentially toxic medication that should only be taken after the person has discussed possible side effects with his or her physician. Although it has been used for many individuals with multiple sclerosis in the United States, Canada, and Europe, its ultimate usefulness in the treatment of MS and its long-term side effects are unknown. Currently, it appears that it can offer benefits to carefully selected individuals. Other immunosuppressants, such as methotrexate, azathioprine (Imuran), and 5-fluorocytosine, pose similar risks, and so there has been little reason to test other combinations of immunosuppressant drugs in people with multiple sclerosis.

Long-Term Suppression of the Immune System

Much of the current research suggests that multiple sclerosis is a disease in which the body's own defense system, the immune system, causes or cooperates in the destruction of the myelin lining of nerves. The immune system is a complex system with many different types of cells interacting to protect the body against disease (Figure 6–2). Certain types of white blood cells, called *suppressor cells,* which ordinarily prevent the immune system from attacking a person's own body, are depressed during MS flare-ups. Whether an immune system gone haywire is a significant factor in the frequency or severity of demyelinating attacks is unknown, but considerable effort has been directed toward suppressing such immune system attacks. Drugs that clearly can suppress various components of the immune system have been available for decades and have found applications in the treatment of diseases of the immune system, such as lymphomas and leukemia. Several of these have been used alone or in combination with other drugs in individuals with multiple sclerosis.

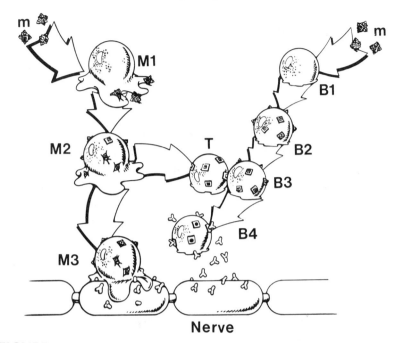

FIGURE 6–2. *Schematic of immune system. Current theories suggest that the agent or virus that causes multiple sclerosis* (m) *interacts with macrophages* (M1) *and B cells* (B1). *This interaction sensitizes the macrophages* (M2) *and B cells* (B2). *T cells* (T) *interact with the sensitized macrophages and in turn stimulate the sensitized B cells* (B3). *The B cells become antibody-producing cells* (B4). *These antibodies and the macrophages* (M3) *attack the myelin sheath of the nerve.*

Drugs other than cyclophosphamide that are effective in suppressing the immune system have been tried many times with very inconsistent results. Azathioprine (Imuran) has been especially popular because it can be taken orally. Administration of this drug every day for weeks or months has not had any definite effect on the course of the disease, but it is routinely given to individuals with multiple sclerosis in several European countries.

Cyclosporine, another drug that inhibits the immune system, has proven exceedingly valuable in preventing rejection of transplanted organs. Because of its effect, cyclosporine was tried in relatively large studies of people with multiple sclerosis. In one study, magnetic resonance imaging of people with multiple sclerosis who took cyclosporine were compared with those of people taking a placebo. The cyclosporine did not significantly affect the course of multiple sclerosis lesions revealed by the MRI scans.

Some physicians urge individuals with progressive multiple sclerosis to continue taking high doses of prednisone, a steroid with an immunosuppressant effect (stops the immune system's functioning). The rationale for this approach is that continuous suppression of immunity will allow fewer flare-ups and less damage from the multiple sclerosis. However, the numerous complications of high-dose steroid use over several months are often as devastating as the multiple sclerosis itself. Consequently, most physicians do not use high-dose prednisone for more than a few days or weeks.

Another problem is that any drug that effectively blocks the body's immune response leaves the person susceptible to infections. Although a person's risk of developing a lethal infection when taking immunosuppressants is small, it is still a reasonable concern when one remembers that multiple sclerosis is not itself a lethal disease. Additional side effects of immunosuppressant drugs include reduction of normal bone marrow activity, with resulting blood clotting disorders or anemia. Intestinal or liver problems develop in some individuals taking these drugs, but in general people with multiple sclerosis tolerate immunosuppressant drugs well. If these drugs improve the long-term outcome of the demyelinating disease, they will be a reasonable treatment option.

Copolymer-1

The synthetic protein Copolymer-1 (Cop-1) has received much attention over the past few years. Preliminary studies suggest that it is more effective than a placebo in reducing the rate of flare-ups. Many researchers believe it reduces long-term disability, but more data are being collected to confirm or refute this idea. Cop-1 is administered by injection under the skin.

Those who believe that Cop-1 is effective think that it works by lessening the immune reactions involved in demyelination. The Cop-1 protein shares properties with some components of myelin. Some researchers have suggested that it works by desensitizing the immune system to elements of myelin, thereby reducing the severity of an immune attack on myelin.

Studies in human subjects have been very limited and injections of this material have yet to produce lasting effects. A study following the progress of people who received Cop-1 did show that some with the relapsing-remitting form of multiple sclerosis improved, but people with the most improvement were those who were least impaired by their disease. This study also supported the claims of some researchers that Copolymer-1 decreases the frequency of attacks experienced by those with mild disability. Unfortunately, this is precisely the group in which the outlook is most unpredictable.

Hyperbaric Oxygen

Oxygen delivered in different ways for different periods of time has been used in efforts to suppress flare-ups and improve the long-term outcome in multiple sclerosis, but it appears to be ineffective (Table 6–2). If an individual is placed in a chamber

TABLE 6–2. Failed Therapies

Hyperbaric oxygen
Cyclosporine
Megavitamins
Vitamin E
Fatty acid supplements
Evening primrose oil
Chiropractic therapy
Acupuncture

with a high concentration of oxygen at pressures exceeding the usual pressure at sea level, an excess of oxygen can be forced into the blood and thereby into the body tissues. This technique, which is called **hyperbaric oxygen therapy,** has been useful in treating infections caused by organisms that cannot tolerate high levels of oxygen, and it has been tried in the management of multiple sclerosis. There are several possible rationales for using hyperbaric oxygen to suppress demyelination, but they are all highly speculative, and the only true measure of the technique's value is the result it produces in people with multiple sclerosis.

Early reports of extraordinary improvement in patients treated with hyperbaric oxygen have not been supported by more extensive studies. Most neurologists are convinced that it has no value in the treatment of multiple sclerosis, but some believe that it can decrease the frequency and severity of flare-ups in selected individuals. Regardless of its effectiveness, there is no reliable information on the long-term effects of hyperbaric oxygen in people with multiple sclerosis. A very real possibility exists that, whether it helps reduce the severity of the demyelinating disease or not, adverse effects of the technique will appear years or decades after its use. The cost of this unproven method is still high, but even if the cost falls or insurance companies agree to pay for treatment sessions, no good evidence has been found that people with multiple sclerosis will profit from the treatment.

Diet

As in any chronic disease, diet is important in minimizing the individual's overall deterioration during a flare-up, but dietary approaches to modifying the frequency and severity of exacerbations have not been effective. Approaches that use extremely large doses of vitamins (megavitamins) have been tried with no success. Because enzymes that use zinc are important in the body's conversion of fatty acids into more useful products, some physicians have recommended foods high in zinc, specifically shellfish and other types of seafood. Adherence to diets rich in specific nutritional factors, such as essential fatty acids (vegetable and fish oils), has been quite disappointing.

Many of the failed therapies based on dietary manipulation grew out of nonmedical fads. The items involved require no special licensing for use, and so this approach to therapy has been more burdened than most by unjustified claims and unsafe regimens. Dietary adjustments are often valuable for individuals with MS, but they should be instituted under the direction of a physician or an experienced nutritionist and should never be misconstrued as a treatment for demyelination or inflammation itself.

Megavitamins

Neurologic problems may develop with diets deficient in some vitamins. This observation and the widespread misconception that vitamins are harmless, regardless of how high a dose is taken, have prompted some individuals to use high doses of vitamins in an effort to treat multiple sclerosis. Unnecessary vitamin supplements do not affect the outcome of multiple sclerosis, but protracted abuse of some vitamins can cause neurologic disease. Because a variety of vitamin regimens have been popular over the past decade, the complications of this approach have become evident.

Thiamine (vitamin B_6) deficiency, a problem common in alcoholic individuals with poor diets, damages nerve cells in both the central and peripheral nervous systems. Because of thiamine's obvious value to the nervous system, many vitamin faddists have proposed taking high daily doses of this vitamin. Such doses, however, can cause numbness in the fingers and toes, unsteadiness in walking, and pins-and-needles sensations.

Vitamin A is important for vision, but an excess can cause increased pressure inside the nervous system, resulting in headaches and impaired vision. This increased pressure is called *pseudotumor cerebri* and can cause permanent damage to vision.

Vitamin B_{12} deficiency causes spinal cord disease with spasticity and weakness, but high doses of this vitamin do not improve any aspect of multiple sclerosis. When a vitamin B_{12} deficiency does occur, it is usually because of a problem with absorbing the vitamin, and so oral supplements do nothing to relieve it.

Known more precisely as *alpha-tocopherol*, vitamin E has gained wide popularity among health food faddists for its purported abilities to improve sex drive and interfere with aging. These claims have been repeatedly discredited, but that has not affected the popularity of this substance. It has also been recommended in some therapy guides for people with multiple sclerosis as a way of reducing flare-ups. The rationale is that alpha-tocopherol interferes with the formation of toxic chemical agents that damage various parts of cells. Although myelin is a cell component, it is not a special target of these toxic agents, but that has not dampened the unfounded enthusiasm vitamin E has enjoyed for several years.

Fatty Acids

Another popular notion is that a low-fat diet, rich in specific fatty acids, such as **primrose oil,** is beneficial. Some physicians have recommended other oils, such as those from sunflower seeds, safflower seeds, corn, and various fishes. The fatty acids usually recommended are those known as *essential fatty acids.* These are substances that, like vitamins, cannot routinely be made by the body and must be included in the diet to avoid malnutrition. The rationale behind taking care to include relatively large portions of these essential fatty acids in the diet is that they are important in nerve and myelin repair and so must be available for the rapid correction of demyelination. Deficiencies in fatty acids may certainly produce nervous system problems, as well as other problems, but it remains unproven that an excess of these foodstuffs will reduce the disability caused by multiple sclerosis.

Evening primrose oil has received special attention because it has a type of fatty acid that is more finished than that found in most animal and vegetable sources. This fatty acid, gamma-linolenic acid, has been claimed to stabilize cell membranes inside and outside the nervous system, as well as to suppress immune system attacks on the nervous system. These claims for the potency of gamma-linolenic and other fatty acids in reducing the frequency and severity of acute exacerbations of the disease are grossly overstated in much of what has been written about multiple sclerosis. Their true value, if any, remains to be established.

Although various dietary regimens have failed to suppress flare-ups or improve remyelination of damaged nerve pathways, careful dietary monitoring is valuable for the person with multiple sclerosis. As discussed in Chapter 7, attention to diet can reduce problems with skin care, bladder disease, and bowel control in individuals with severe MS. A well-balanced diet is vital in any treatment plan intended to reduce the complications of multiple sclerosis.

Nonmedical Approaches

Every person with multiple sclerosis is burdened by stories from family and friends of miraculous cures. Faith healers, snake oil merchants, gurus, and yoga experts inevitably have the cure to all problems. What superficially appear to be harmless and inexpensive approaches invariably prove damaging and costly.

Despite claims by their practitioners, chiropractic therapy and acupuncture are ineffective therapies. Some people may feel better for a short time during manipulation, massage, or puncture, but none of these benefits lasts more than minutes or hours, and most can be tied to a placebo effect. Although these techniques are ineffective, they are not free of complications. Muscle contusions and ligament tears can develop with chiropractic therapy and infections can occur with acupuncture if poor technique is used.

There is a great deal of pressure to try these unconventional therapies, but the person with multiple sclerosis should resist that pressure. In many families, ignoring advice is considered an insult to the person offering it, but the interests of the person with multiple sclerosis are best served if he or she simply acknowledges the recommendation and ignores it.

Other Approaches

Many other types of treatment have been applied to the management of multiple sclerosis, but few have shown much promise. Treatment plans introduced over the past few decades have sought either to limit the immune response that appears to be so important in demyelination or to enhance remyelination, which is vital to recovery of normal nerve function. Whatever approach has been tried, the researchers have had to consider their results in the context of the side effects that their techniques produce.

Thymectomy

The **thymus** is a gland that sits in the middle of the chest, just above the heart (Figure 6–3). It is important in the operation of certain elements of the immune system and has consequently attracted the interest of researchers trying to suppress the immune system elements active in demyelination. White blood cells called **T cells** or T lymphocytes interact with the thymus as they mature. In some autoimmune diseases, such as the muscle disease myasthenia gravis, removal of the thymus has improved the course of the disease. Because of this experience and because T cells appear to play a major role in demyelination, some investigators have removed the thymus glands from people with multiple sclerosis. The results have not been consistent, and the practice is still not considered a reasonable therapy except as part of a research study.

Plasmapheresis

One technique that allows the removal of specific elements from the blood is called *plasmapheresis*. In one variation of this technique, called *lymphocytapheresis,* lymphocytes are removed from the blood. The objective in using this procedure for people with multiple sclerosis is to remove the white blood cells that appear to

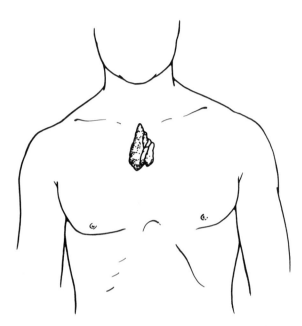

FIGURE 6–3. *The thymus is a small gland, located in the center of the chest, with a major role in the immune system.*

be a part of the demyelination process. This produces a very transient change in blood composition, because mechanisms in the bone marrow and elsewhere will immediately attempt to correct the deficiency that has been artificially produced.

Plasmapheresis must be repeated several times to truly affect the composition of the blood. With each treatment, the subject is exposed to some risk of infection simply by virtue of the type of equipment that is used and the procedures that are followed. This is generally viewed as a safe technique, however, and it has found considerable application in a variety of blood disorders.

Its effectiveness in multiple sclerosis is controversial, but the consensus is that it does not substantially affect the course or severity of multiple sclerosis. As the technique is refined and blood elements can be more selectively extracted, the technique may prove to be much more useful than it currently appears to be.

Thoracic Duct Drainage

White blood cells (lymphocytes) can be depleted by techniques other than lymphocytapheresis. One method is thoracic duct drainage. The thoracic duct is a major conduit for the return of white blood cells to the bloodstream. Thoracic duct drainage is time-consuming and difficult. It also allows little specificity in the type of lymphocyte removed. Although a few investigators have reported good results with this method, most physicians are unconvinced.

Treatment Perspectives

No thoroughly satisfactory treatment of acute or chronic disease is currently available. As discussed in Chapter 11, much research is being done to find safe and effective treatments, but truly promising results have been in short supply. Until safe and effective therapies are fully developed and tested, the person with multiple sclerosis should avoid fads. Even the most benign interventions such as radical diets, spinal manipulation, acupuncture, and vitamin supplements, can cause nervous system damage when applied to the person with multiple sclerosis. People with MS certainly should participate in experimental studies if they are interested, but all experimental therapy programs should be conducted by physicians at medical institutions, not by individuals with secret concoctions.

Treatment of Common Problems

There are many effective treatments for the problems that develop with multiple sclerosis. Even in cases with severe complications, many of the symptoms can be reversed or lessened with conventional medical approaches. Drugs will help with many of the chronic problems that appear in people with severe disease, and modifications in diet or lifestyle may suffice to eliminate symptoms in those with mild disease. With more extensive disturbances of nervous system function, surgical procedures may be useful, but this will be true for a small proportion of the people affected by multiple sclerosis.

Routine follow-up visits with a physician are an essential part of every treatment plan. Some physicians and most people with multiple sclerosis believe that mild symptoms, such as transient weakness or rapidly resolving loss of vision, during the first few months of disease indicate that future complications will be mild, but this is not true. Severe neurologic disease causes little trouble during the first year it produces symptoms. Consequently, careful medical follow-up is necessary, regardless of how well the individual looks and feels early in the course of the illness.

Most of the signs and symptoms of multiple sclerosis can be minimized, compensated for, or corrected with appropriate medical treatment, environmental modifications, or physical therapy. In designing a treatment program, the principal physician and therapist must consider all of a person's abilities and disabilities. What is appropriate for the individual with multiple sclerosis will be determined not only by the severity of the signs and symptoms present, but also by their durations and complications.

Relieving Spasticity

Changes in muscle stiffness may be transient, but if they persist for more than a few months, they warrant treatment. Even when the person has relatively little limb stiffness or spasticity, the awkwardness or clumsiness produced by this disturbance of muscle tone deserves treatment (Table 7–1). Exercise and physical therapy may help to reduce the discomfort caused by mild spasticity, but most people will require additional treatment with medications. If spasticity persists for years and produces other complications, such as pressure sores and frozen joints, surgical interruption of the nerve pathways sustaining the abnormal tension in the muscle may be helpful.

TABLE 7–1. Therapy for Spasticity

Physical therapy
Stretching exercises
Antispasticity agents

Physical Therapy

Much of the discomfort and disability that develops with mild spasticity results from injuries to joints. Muscle actions must be well coordinated to align the joints properly as a limb is moved. One of the benefits of physical therapy for the person with mild spasticity is that it exercises the joints in proper alignment and provides stress-reducing aids to minimize the trauma to joints. Stretching and strengthening exercises that will maximize the usefulness of the limb and minimize the trauma occurring at the joints can be devised by an experienced therapist.

Some of the problems faced during routine activities can be solved by muscle retraining. Individuals with significant spasticity and clonus (rapid alternation of muscle contraction and relaxation, causing jerkiness) may experience much difficulty on trying to rise from a sitting position, but modifying the procedure used for getting up may be more effective than efforts to reduce the spasticity. Many find that getting up is simpler if they place both feet flat on the floor when they try to stand, rather than rising from the toes as most people automatically do.

For some individuals, mechanical aids are as helpful as or more helpful than exercises in preserving joint structures. If poor control of the muscles in lifting the foot up or poor relaxation of the muscles in putting the foot down produces a **foot drop** (Figure 7–1), much discomfort and joint disease can be eliminated by using a splint to passively realign the ankle. This splint can be made of lightweight plastic with a design that allows it to slip into ordinary shoes and remain concealed under ankle-length clothing (Figure 7–2).

The person with poor spine alignment may avoid much back pain and curvature by using properly designed corsets or braces. Excessive dependence on braces should be avoided, however, because they allow muscles essential for normal posture to weaken. When used under the direction of a skilled physiatrist or physical therapist, braces can reduce the pain and increase mobility. Exercise programs formulated by an experienced

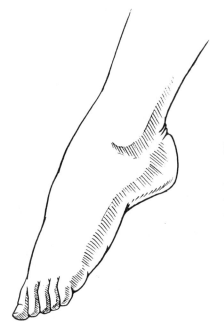

FIGURE 7–1. *Footdrop: Weakness in muscles dorsiflexing the foot can prevent the foot from coming off the ground, causing the individual to drag that foot.*

physiatrist are also usually helpful in minimizing the effects of spasticity.

Drug Treatment

Several drugs are widely used to reduce muscle stiffness or limb spasticity. Finding out which is most appropriate for an individual may require some trial and error, but there are a few that are often useful (Table 7–2). Some of these agents act in the nervous system, some act directly on the muscle, and some act at unidentified sites. To be effective, an agent need not eliminate the spasticity itself. Drugs that appear to do little more than reduce the inflammation associated with recurrent trauma to poorly aligned joints may reduce a person's pain and disability considerably.

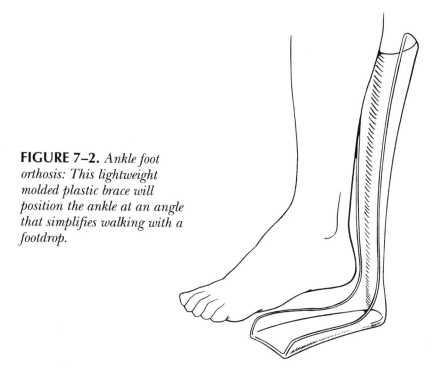

FIGURE 7–2. *Ankle foot orthosis: This lightweight molded plastic brace will position the ankle at an angle that simplifies walking with a footdrop.*

TABLE 7–2. Treatment of Spasticity

Antispasticity Drugs
Baclofen (Lioresal)
Dantrolene sodium (Dantrium)
Muscle Relaxants
Diazepam (Valium)
Chlordiazepoxide (Librium)
Methocarbamol (Robaxin)
Other Muscle Relaxants
Anti-inflammatory Drugs
Nerve Blocks
Nerve Destruction

Baclofen

Baclofen (Lioresal) is a drug developed specifically to combat spasticity. It appears to act in the spinal cord to relieve limb spasticity. It is usually well-tolerated and so it has found wide application. This drug is of most use when the spasticity caused by the demyelination is severe, but limb strength is still fairly good. If the limb is weak and spastic, eliminating the spasticity may do little to improve its usefulness. A weak leg that is kept in a straight position by spasticity is easier to walk on than a weak limb that has normal or decreased muscle tone.

There are individuals, however, who have poor limb strength and severe spasticity for whom relief of the spasticity is important. These include people whose limbs have assumed postures that interfere with routine care and may result in pressure sores and contractures. In some cases, severe spasticity causes uncontrollable pain. Relieving the spasticity becomes an essential step in pain management.

The usual dose of baclofen is about 10 mg orally three to four times daily, but most patients must start by taking a dose of 5 to 10 mg daily and gradually increasing the total daily dose over the course of several weeks. Starting at a full dose usually causes drowsiness. Some individuals also complain of nausea; many experience weakness.

After days or weeks at a low dose, the affected person can usually tolerate a much higher dose with little sedation or weakness. Some people with multiple sclerosis will benefit from baclofen doses in excess of 50 mg daily, but exposing someone to such high doses is only appropriate when he or she shows a response at lower doses and exhibits a high level of tolerance for the drug. The physician must check blood chemistries every few weeks or months while a person is taking this drug, because it does cause changes in kidney function in susceptible individuals. This is not a common problem, however.

For individuals with severe spasticity in the legs or poor tolerance of orally administered baclofen, an infusion pump may be useful. This device automatically pumps minute doses of baclofen into the spinal fluid surrounding the spinal cord. The infusion apparatus may be left in place for long periods, but regular follow-up visits with a physician are essential to minimize complications of this device.

Interactions between drugs must be considered whenever someone takes more than one drug. The physician prescribing baclofen or other antispasticity agents should be advised of all medications that a person uses, even nonprescription drugs or vitamins. Reactions to baclofen, such as sedation or urinary retention, may resolve completely when the other medications are reduced or eliminated.

Dantrolene Sodium

Dantrolene sodium (Dantrium) and deanol (Deaner) are alternatives to baclofen in the management of spasticity. Deanol is no longer available in the United States, but dantrolene sodium is still popular. Sedation may be a problem with either of these two drugs, just as with baclofen. Occasionally, individuals may have liver disturbances or allergic reactions. None of these antispasticity drugs can be taken except under the continuing supervision of a physician.

Muscle Relaxants

Many drugs referred to as muscle relaxants probably have little or no direct effect on muscles, but that does not mean that they are not useful in managing complaints of muscle stiffness. A family of drugs called *benzodiazepines* has been used extensively in people with multiple sclerosis and spasticity. The more familiar members of this family are diazepam (Valium) and chlordiazepoxide (Librium). An increasing number of physicians are also using clonazepam (Klonopin), another benzodiazepine. Precisely how these drugs affect the tension in muscles or, in fact, whether they do affect it is less important than that they do improve mobility for many people with complaints of muscle stiffness. The most common side effect with these drugs is lethargy, a problem that may appear even at low doses. Unpredictable sensitivity reactions also are a problem with these drugs, as they are for all drugs.

Diazepam, chlordiazepoxide, or clonazepam may be used in combination with baclofen or dantrolene. Most will find that such combinations make them very sleepy, but a few will have less spasticity with the combination than with either drug taken alone. Before using these drugs with other medications, a person should ask the physician about possible interactions.

Despite widely publicized reports of dependence on these medications once they are used on a regular basis, addiction is rare and usually only develops in individuals predisposed to becoming dependent on a variety of substances that are not typically addicting. Ordinarily, a person with multiple sclerosis will not become addicted to these drugs, but after taking them each day for several months he or she will notice restlessness and insomnia if the drug is omitted for a day or two. These withdrawal effects pass uneventfully after a few days off the medication.

Methocarbamol (Robaxin) is one of the more popular non-benzodiazepine drugs used as a muscle relaxant. Whether it actually relaxes muscles can be debated, but it certainly makes some individuals less aware of limb stiffness. How it works has not been determined, and for whom it will be effective is unpredictable. Most will find that it does little more than sedate them, but some will find that it reduces the discomfort associated with chronic spasticity and recurrent spasms.

Anti-inflammatory Drugs

Several over-the-counter and prescription drugs that reduce inflammation are helpful in managing the discomfort associated with spasticity. Some of the pain that those with spasticity and muscle spasms feel is actually from tendon strains, joint injuries, and pulled ligaments. This type of injury develops slowly and so is not recognized as a problem separate from the neurologic problem itself. Medications that reduce the inflammation associated with these injuries usually reduce the pain that it causes.

Ibuprofen (Motrin, Advil, Nuprin), naproxen (Naprosyn, Anaprox, Alleve), piroxicam (Feldene), and diflunisal (Dolobid) are all nonsteroidal anti-inflammatory drugs that are commonly used by individuals with painful spasticity. Who will profit from using them is unpredictable. Most cause some stomach or intestinal discomfort, and so individuals with gastrointestinal problems should use such medications cautiously.

Illicit Drugs

Some people with multiple sclerosis experiment with illegally purchased or illicitly produced drugs, but this is unwise. Marijuana (THC) and cocaine or crack may improve one's sense of well-being transiently, but both carry high risks of complications. Marijuana is often contaminated with herbicides or pesticides, and cocaine or crack is usually adulterated with amphetamines (speed) or anesthetic agents (Novocaine, Xylocaine). These unwanted additives can cause reactions ranging from problems with breathing to irregular heartbeats. The advantages of these drugs have not been systemically studied in individuals with multiple sclerosis, and so it is impossible to know if pure agents would be useful in managing problems like spasticity. The addictiveness of cocaine makes it an unattractive option even if it did prove effective against some symptoms.

Nerve Destruction

Spasticity is a result of brain or spinal cord disease, but it requires muscle contractions to produce the abnormal stiffness. The muscles are stimulated by inappropriate messages delivered along the nerves to the muscles. If all the nerves to a muscle are cut, it becomes limp and paralyzed. Without the inappropriate nerve activity that occurs in spasticity, there can be no spasticity. This means that spasticity can be eliminated by cutting the nerves to the muscles involved. This is a drastic measure that should never be considered unless intractable spasticity has made a limb useless for several years and the spasticity itself is producing serious complications, such as infected pressure sores. This procedure is discussed below in the section on managing complications of severe disease. A baclofen infusion pump is an alternative to nerve destruction in some cases.

Managing Bladder Disorders

Problems with bladder control range from occasional dribbling when the bladder feels full to total loss of control with no warning. For most individuals with multiple sclerosis, the major concern is that the bladder will empty unexpectedly and cause embarrassment or ruin clothing. For people with only minor bladder control problems, loss of urine during sleep, a condition called *enuresis,* is more common than daytime incontinence but is less likely to prompt medical attention. Bed-wetting is a much less public and less easily detected problem than daytime incontinence, but it can cause domestic stress if the person does not sleep alone. The need to repeatedly clean urine-soaked sheets and mattresses invariably produces a strain in family or intimate relationships.

Although incontinence can have great impact on the affected individual and his or her family, for many people the management of incontinence is quite simple. If it occurs only at night, it often stops with little more than avoiding late-evening drinks. Reducing the amount of fluid the body must handle during sleep reduces the amount that accumulates in the bladder at night. Those who fail to do well with this altered routine may achieve full control with medication that inhibits bladder emptying at night. If problems with bladder control cannot be managed with medication, surgical or mechanical intervention is needed to avoid serious complications, such as repeated bladder infections and progressive kidney disease. One of the dangers with incontinence is frequent bladder infections. Problems in the bladder can and often do find their way back upstream to the kidneys even if the individual is healthy enough to limit spread of infections outside of the urinary tract. Because of these dangers, a physician should regularly monitor bladder and kidney function to make sure that no treatment is needed.

Anyone with bladder control problems is susceptible to urinary tract infections. The routine warning of discomfort on urination that alerts people with pain perception to a bladder infection may not be available to the person with multiple sclerosis. Spinal cord disease that interferes with normal bladder function is likely also to interfere with normal bladder and urinary outlet sensation. This means that those people with bladder disorders caused by multiple sclerosis must be careful to look for changes in the appearance of their urine, such as blood, pus, or just discoloration, to minimize the risk of a bladder infection.

Mechanical and Dietary Strategies

The person with only occasional incontinence may need little more than absorbent undergarments. Bulky diapers are not necessary. Highly absorbent, leak-proof pads are available and will limit the damage caused by a minor lapse in bladder control. Whatever precautions can be taken to reduce the amount of fluid that must be handled by the bladder should be used routinely. Fluid restriction is wise before activities, such as sports and sexual intercourse, in which loss of bladder control is especially likely. During sleep, the bladder empties because of prolonged filling; during sports and sexual activity, direct pressure on the bladder may trigger emptying (Table 7–3).

Some people unknowingly stress the bladder's ability to retain urine by drinking fluids high in irritants or diuretics, agents that increase the rate at which water is eliminated from the body. Caffeinated drinks, such as cola, tea, and coffee, increase bladder output and irritability. Alcohol also drives water out of the body and increases the amount of fluid that must accumulate in the bladder each hour. These substances all produce incontinence by

TABLE 7–3. Sources of Stress on the Bladder
Sports activity
Sexual activity
Diuretics
Cola drinks
Tea
Coffee
Alcoholic beverages

the extra demands they make on the bladder, even if the actual additional demand is quite small.

Drugs to Regulate Bladder Empyting

If treatment for a bladder disorder is needed, it will usually consist of getting the bladder to empty more effectively or to empty less prematurely. Some drugs interfere with bladder emptying by blocking reflexes in the spinal cord or in the wall of the bladder itself. One class of drugs that will do this is called *anticholinergic*. Of the many anticholinergic drugs used, two of the safest are imipramine (Tofranil), a widely used antidepressant that has long been used to manage bed-wetting in children, and oxybutynin chloride (Ditropan), a drug that acts directly on the neural regulation of bladder contractions.

For many people with multiple sclerosis, a single evening dose of 100 mg of imipramine suppresses bladder activity enough to provide for a relatively carefree day. Oxybutynin is given in 5 mg doses two to four times daily. With both of these drugs, the individual should watch for harmful side effects. These drugs interfere with nervous system activity that increases bladder emptying, but they also affect other functions of the nervous system, such as heat regulation and gastrointestinal function, causing hot flashes and diarrhea in sensitive individuals.

Catheterization

With severe bladder disturbances, drugs to regulate bladder emptying may not suffice. Other techniques must be adopted to empty the bladder, the simplest being the introduction of a catheter, a thin tube that can pass through the urinary tract into the bladder. Passing this catheter into the bladder provides an outlet for urine trapped there. The force driving the urine through the catheter is the tone of muscles in the bladder or in the wall of the abdomen overlying the bladder. If these muscles have little tone, the individual can force urine out by simply pressing on the abdominal wall. Once the catheter has eliminated the block to the free outflow of urine, the bladder can be emptied.

This technique, called *catheterization,* is more than 1000 years old. It requires no complex equipment and is especially simple for women with bladder emptying problems. The longer distance between the bladder neck and the exit point for urine passed through the penis makes the use of a catheter a bit more complicated for men. If the prostate gland, which only men have, is enlarged, the job of threading a catheter into the bladder can be very difficult. Despite such problems, most men can be trained to perform self-catheterization if their hand coordination is fair.

Frequent catheterization is the safest approach for the woman with bladder control problems who fails to benefit from medication. Most women can be trained to catheterize themselves. If a man can be trained to perform the relatively difficult technique of self-catheterization safely, this procedure is usually preferable to leaving a catheter (called a *Foley catheter*) in the bladder or a condom with a draining catheter (called a *Texas catheter*) on the penis. Fewer infections develop when a person with MS learns to insert and remove a catheter even though he or she does not sterilize the catheter before using it.

Self-catheterization is most effective in managing incontinence if it is done on a regular schedule. The affected person can carry a catheter during the day and introduce it into the bladder after simply washing and lubricating it. After the bladder empties, the tube can be removed, washed, and stored for later use. A new catheter is not needed each time the bladder is emptied. The only facility needed for this procedure is a reasonably clean bathroom with running water.

Infection Control

Individuals who abruptly develop urinary incontinence with no other signs of a flare-up of their multiple sclerosis may have a bladder infection. Infections usually produce burning on urination, foul-smelling urine, or urine discolored by blood or clouded by pus. Incontinence may be the principal or only sign of infection in individuals with marginally effective bladder control. Women are especially susceptible because of the short length of the urethra, the connection between the bladder and the urinary outlet. In men, the urethra must traverse the entire length of the penis, so an infection is less likely to find its way to the bladder.

Urinalysis

Whenever a bladder infection is suspected, the urine should be checked for bacteria and signs of inflammation. White blood cells, some red blood cells, and other material not usually found in the urine can be readily detected on a microscopic examination and routine chemical testing of the fluid, a procedure called *urinalysis*. The bacteria causing the infection can be grown in the laboratory and identified at the time of this analysis. Identification of the responsible bacteria is important because it will determine which antibiotic is most appropriate for treating the infection.

Antibiotics

If the microscopic examination of the urine reveals infection, most doctors will start antibiotic treatment even before the bacteria have been identified. Drugs commonly used include ampicillin, Bactrim, and Septra. Bactrim and Septra are combinations of antibiotics, rather than a single drug. Most patients tolerate these drugs well, but some will be allergic to the medication, and alternatives must be found. People with allergies to penicillin will usually be allergic to ampicillin. A commonly used alternative drug in such cases is cephalexin (Keflex).

Prevention of Urinary Tract Infections

Individuals with susceptibility to infection can take several measures to reduce the risk. For women, cleaning the groin area around the urinary outlet is very important. Mild soap and water are adequate; harsh detergents should not be used because they can cause vaginal irritation, as well as urethral irritation. Most bladder infections have difficulty thriving in very acidic urine, and so it is often helpful to acidify the urine by drinking prune or cranberry juice (Table 7–4). Eating foods high in protein, such as meat and poultry, will also help to acidify the urine. Orange, grapefruit, and tomato juice all reduce the acidity of the urine, so they should not be drunk when infection is likely. These juices have vitamin C, ascorbic acid, which will help reduce the risk of bladder infection, but this vitamin is available as a vitamin supplement and is better taken in that form if frequent bladder infections become a problem. Vitamin C should not be taken in a dose of greater than 500 mg at one time or more often than four times daily.

For some individuals with multiple sclerosis, continuous antibiotic treatment may be necessary to avoid frequent urinary tract infections. Long-term administration of combination antibiotics, such as Septra and Bactrim, may be the only approach that successfully blocks the development of overwhelming bladder infections.

TABLE 7–4. Agents Affecting Urine Acidity

Increasing Acidity	Decreasing Acidity
Prune juice	Orange juice
Cranberry juice	Grapefruit juice
Meat	Tomato Juice
Poultry	

Long-term treatment with a single antibiotic should not be used routinely to deal with the risk of infection because organisms will usually develop resistance to an agent to which they are constantly exposed, but if bladder infections reappear frequently, such treatment is helpful. Treatment with antibiotics requires ongoing supervision by a urologist or other competent physician.

Treating Bowel Problems

People with multiple sclerosis do not usually develop serious problems with stomach or intestinal activity, but some problems do result from inactivity and medication side effects. Constipation often develops in people who, either because of pain or weakness, cannot be active. The usual approach to this problem is laxatives, but that type of intervention is far from ideal. What is more reasonable and less disturbing to intestinal function is a change in diet and a concerted effort to increase daily activity (Table 7–5).

Dietary Precautions

Additional fluids may help considerably, especially if fruit juices are the major source of the additional fluids. At least two quarts of

---

TABLE 7–5. Managing Constipation

Increase daily fluid intake.
Add fresh fruits and vegetables to the diet.
Increase bulk and fiber by eating bran cereals and whole grain breads.
Eat 2 tablespoons of 100% bran in the morning.
Take a bulk laxative (for instance, mucilloid of psyllium seed, Metamucil) at night.
Avoid peas, beans, and sugar.
Take 100 mg of dioctyl sodium sulfosuccinate (Colace) twice daily if diet fails.

fluid should be a regular part of the daily diet. Increasing fluid intake may be impractical, however, if the individual also has a problem with urinary incontinence. Fluid restrictions designed to improve bladder control may exacerbate constipation, so other changes in the diet must be attempted.

Loading the diet with high-fiber foods and unprocessed fruits should help to avoid constipation. Bran cereals and whole-grain breads will increase the bulk and fiber in the diet and improve the ease of bowel movements. Bran is available as a powder or granular substance to add to cereals. Eating the bran alone is difficult because it tastes unpleasantly bland.

Some naturally occurring substances, such as a component of psyllium seeds used in Metamucil, are effective bulk laxatives and can increase the regularity of bowel movements if they are used on a daily basis. Sugar, peas, beans, and other foods that produce substantial intestinal gas should be avoided because they can make the individual with constipation even more uncomfortable.

Medications for Constipation

If this strictly dietary approach fails, an agent that simply pulls water into the intestines without causing irritation may be effective. Several medications work in this way; one of the more commonly prescribed substances is dioctyl sodium sulfosuccinate (Colace). A dosage of 100 to 200 mg of this drug daily usually ensures regular bowel activity. Many over-the-counter laxatives also are safe and reliable when used infrequently. Milk of magnesia taken at night will usually provide relief from constipation the following day. More rapidly acting agents, such as magnesium citrate, are widely available, but they are very irritating to the gastrointestinal tract and should not be used unless milder agents have failed to relieve the constipation.

Many people become worried when they fail to have a bowel movement regularly, but there is nothing intrinsically dangerous about not having a bowel movement every day. When severe impaction occurs, it can usually be relieved with a soap-suds or

Fleets enema. In extreme cases, manual disimpaction may be necessary, but this type of intervention should be attempted only by experienced personnel.

Treatment for Fecal Incontinence

Fecal incontinence, the inability to keep from soiling oneself with stool, usually does not develop in people with multiple sclerosis. With loss of sensation and strength below the level of the waist, however, some individuals become unable to control their bowel movements. Drugs used to manage other problems, such as the antibiotics used to manage bladder infections, may irritate the intestines and cause fecal incontinence in those who still have relatively good bowel control. Whenever fecal incontinence develops, another cause should be sought before multiple sclerosis alone is blamed.

There is currently no medication that will inhibit this bowel activity, but for many the problem is short-lived. For those few in whom bowel incontinence persists, dietary practices may allow the development of a rhythm that greatly simplifies care. Shortly after a meal, the intestinal activity reflexively increases. A bowel movement is likely to occur at that time, especially if a regular schedule is adopted for meals. Placing the person on a commode or bedpan at that time may avoid accidental soiling. Those with fecal incontinence face the same problems of skin care faced by individuals with bladder incontinence.

In rare cases, bowel incontinence becomes so substantial a problem that the individual may choose to have the intestines surgically revised so that they empty into a bag on the front of the abdomen. This procedure, called a *colostomy,* is usually not necessary, but people with years of bowel problems may prefer this revision to living in diapers. A colostomy should never be done unless the coping techniques above have been followed faithfully and the bowel incontinence has been a problem for over a year, simply because poor bowel control, like other problems developing with multiple sclerosis, may abate in time.

Controlling Pain

Any attempt to control pain must first consider what the actual cause of the pain is. If the person has an infection or a sprained ligament, antibiotic treatment or splinting may do much more to relieve the discomfort than will pain killers. If a joint is dislocated, it must be realigned. If collapse of a vertebral body in the spine is causing the pain, weight-bearing on the weak bone must be eliminated. Even when the pain is typical of that caused by demyelinating disease, such as the shooting facial pains of trigeminal neuralgia, a person and his or her physician cannot assume that there is no local problem causing the discomfort. If there is no local problem, multiple sclerosis may be the basis for the pain. The abnormal sensations that develop with damage to central nervous system pathways for sensation can be quite disabling.

A variety of approaches have been used for managing pain that develops because of demyelinating disease (Table 7–6). These include using analgesic (that is, pain-killing) drugs, but most of the drugs that are useful are not pain killers. Other mechanisms for modifying sensation, such as electrical stimula-

---

TABLE 7–6. Techniques for Pain Management

Analgesics
Tricyclic antidepressants
Other drugs
TENS
Acupuncture
Steroid injections
Physical therapy
Nerve destruction
Dorsal column stimulators
Spinal cord surgery

tion of a nerve, acupuncture, and steroid injections into nerves, have been used with questionable effectiveness and safety. Perhaps the safest and often the most effective approach to pain is physical therapy (see Chapter 10).

Certain types of pain are especially common in individuals with multiple sclerosis. As already mentioned, the pain associated with optic neuritis may respond dramatically to steroids, the most commonly used being prednisone. The shooting facial pains of trigeminal neuralgia are also more common in multiple sclerosis than in other types of neurologic disease. Carbamazepine (Tegretol) is generally considered the drug of choice for this disorder and is discussed in more detail later. Abnormal sensations that seem to arise because of central nervous system damage often respond to tricyclic antidepressants, such as imipramine (Tofranil) and amitriptyline (Elavil).

Drug Therapy

When there is no obvious cause for pain, burning, tingling, or electrical sensations, most physicians will try managing the problem with mild pain killers (nonnarcotic analgesics). If this fails, as it often does, drugs that interfere with the handling of sensory information in the central nervous system are usually effective. Consequently, it is wrong to increase the strength and dosage of pain killers so that the individual is eventually using high doses of addictive drugs, such as morphine, meperidine (Demerol), or methadone. Some of the more commonly used nonanalgesic drugs are carbamazepine (Tegretol), phenytoin (Dilantin, Epanutin), and imipramine (Tofranil). Each of these drugs may cause complications, but they are generally safer than narcotic analgesics.

Carbamazepine (Tegretol)

Carbamazepine was developed as an antiepileptic medication, but was recognized soon after its development to be effective against the pain of trigeminal neuralgia in many people. It is usually given in doses of 200 to 400 mg each three to four times daily. Most people feel tired or nauseated when they first start on a large dose of this drug, so a smaller dose is used when the drug is introduced. Some people cannot use this drug because they develop rashes or blood reactions, but most find that they can tolerate the drug when they are on a dose that does not sedate or nauseate them.

Carbamazepine must be taken on a regular basis to be effective. It will have little or no effect on pain if it is only taken on the day the person has discomfort. To be effective, a steady level of the drug must be present in the bloodstream. The physician prescribing this medication will check the blood level of the drug every few weeks or months to be sure that an excessive amount is not accumulating in the body. Most will also periodically check blood counts and blood chemistries. A drop in the white blood cell count (called *leukopenia*) often occurs with this drug, but it is usually not a reason for stopping the drug unless the white cell count reaches dangerously low levels.

Phenytoin (Dilantin, Epanutin)

Phenytoin is also an antiepileptic medication that is more widely recognized for its ability to suppress abnormal heart activity than for its effect on pain. It is usually taken as a 100-mg capsule three to four times daily, but it can be taken just once a day as a dose of 300 to 400 mg. It must be taken on a regular basis, rather than when pain occurs, for it to be effective. Pain problems are usually not affected by the drug until the individual has taken it for several days.

Because phenytoin is absorbed slowly into the body, individuals may start on a full dose with little risk of unpleasant effects; those that may occur include sedation, clumsiness, unsteady walking, and slurred speech. Some people are allergic to the drug or have idiosyncratic blood reactions to it; such reactions require immediate withdrawal of the drug. The slow accumulation of significant amounts of the drug in the blood results in a very gradual change in the amount of pain experienced. The amount of drug in the blood can and should be monitored by the physician. Checking it every few months will ensure that the individual does not develop an excessive level.

Imipramine (Tofranil)

Imipramine has already been discussed because of its use in the management of bladder control problems. It belongs to the family of drugs called *tricyclics*. These include amitriptyline and other antidepressant drugs, many of which are also useful in relieving the pain that develops with demyelinating disease. Its principal side effects are sedation, retention of urine, and dry mouth.

Tricyclic antidepressants accumulate very slowly in the blood. Those taking this medication for pain management will usually not see any results until they have taken it every day for more than a week. To be effective, the drugs must be taken on a continuing basis.

Treatment Guidelines

Why any of these drugs makes a difference in pain syndromes is unknown, but it is clear that they do diminish discomfort in people with disturbed central nervous system function. The patient taking any of these drugs should be given the lowest effective dose possible, and when symptoms have been relieved for weeks, the drug should be withdrawn slowly to see whether the problem has completely resolved or if the drug is simply masking the symptom. Any of these drugs can be used for years if needed. Both carbamazepine and phenytoin are routinely given to individuals with epilepsy for years at a time with little long-term change caused by the drug. Imipramine is a widely prescribed antidepressant. People with multiple sclerosis can be treated with this for months, if not years, without harm, as long as blood tests are routinely performed to check for adverse reactions.

Recent insights into the nervous system chemicals that modify pain recognition may provide new classes of drugs for managing pain in the future. The endorphins, for instance, seem to act in much the same way as morphine, but they are naturally occurring substances in the brain and spinal cord. What side effects will develop with administration of these drugs to people with chronic pain remains to be determined.

Transcutaneous Electric Nerve Stimulation (TENS)

Many abnormal sensations can be blocked by applying an electric current to a nerve controlling the area from which the abnormal sensations originate. This electric stimulation can be applied through the skin, in which case the procedure is called *transcutaneous electric nerve stimulation,* or TENS. Its effectiveness for many different pain syndromes is clear. That it is safe is not clear, at least in the case of multiple sclerosis.

Many physicians believe that TENS worsens the symptoms of multiple sclerosis in those who receive this treatment for pain. The individual's own experience with the technique is more important than any general rules, however. If pain persists after use of more conventional approaches, TENS may provide an effective alternative. It should be used only if the treatments are supervised by an experienced physician.

Unconventional Techniques

Often people who get no relief from pain despite traditional medical approaches turn to more unconventional techniques. Many of these techniques are simply quackery, but others do help. The person with a constant pins-and-needles sensation on his arm may find that bathing the arm in warm water provides relief. Stretching exercises or exertion with a limb may relieve chronic (that is, long-lasting) pain, at least temporarily. There has been no reliable assessment of the value of acupuncture in the management of pain caused by central nervous system demyelination, but it has been of value to some individuals. Aggressive treatment of pain with spinal cord surgery or electric stimulation of the dorsal column of the spinal cord may be effective, but such treatments are quite dangerous and usually unnecessary. They are discussed in more detail later in this chapter.

Chiropractic therapy has been popular in the United States for many decades, but it has no place in the management of multiple sclerosis. The abnormal muscle activity that may occur with multiple sclerosis poses resistance to movement that chiropractors are not trained to manage. Excessive spinal manipulation can cause problems ranging from muscle injuries to joint damage.

Treating Fatigue

With any nervous system disorder, the affected person often notices that he or she tires more rapidly. This is true whether the injury is a concussion after an automobile accident or demyelination from multiple sclerosis. Attempts to manage the fatigue that appears with multiple sclerosis have been frustrated by the unpredictability of the symptom. It is likely to come and go whether the affected person receives treatment or not.

Whenever fatigue becomes a major problem, the individual should have a thorough medical reevaluation. Fatigue cannot be assumed to arise from the central nervous system disease simply because an individual has multiple sclerosis (Table 7–7). Chronic infection, anemia, or even inapparent fractures may all be the source of the fatigue. A thorough physical examination with laboratory studies of the blood count and urine components may reveal a correctable basis for the fatigue. Daytime fatigue often proves to be from sleeplessness associated with depression, pain, or drug reactions.

If the central nervous system disease is the sole basis for the

TABLE 7–7. Causes of Fatigue

Demyelination
Sleep deprivation
Infection
Fractures
Anemia
Kidney disease

fatigue, the person should adjust his or her level of activity to avoid exhaustion. This does not mean that he or she should become inactive. As much exercise and intellectual activity as is tolerable should be performed on a regular basis.

Stimulants

Several drugs have shown some promise in managing fatigue over the long term. Amantadine (Symmetrel), an antiviral agent that is widely used in the treatment of Parkinson's disease, has also been of value in some patients with multiple sclerosis. In both Parkinson's disease and multiple sclerosis, the drug is presumed to affect chemical transmitters in the brain. It is usually taken as a single 100-mg tablet once or twice a day. The value of this drug usually lessens after a few months, but intermittent treatment may help some people. Why this drug is effective is unknown. Side effects are rare and are usually little more than allergic reactions or mood disturbances.

Amphetamines (Dexedrine, speed) and many other types of stimulants, such as caffeine and Dexatrim, are not helpful. These drugs overburden an already damaged nervous system and should be strictly avoided. Cocaine is often viewed as a less harmful stimulant, but it too is inadvisable. The central nervous system effect of cocaine in the person with multiple sclerosis is unpredictable, and the drug is addicting. Because cocaine is still an illegal drug in most countries, adulteration of the cocaine with other substances places the person with demyelinating disease at special risk. In the United States, cocaine is often mixed with amphetamines. Regular use results in addiction. Even occasional use may produce potentially fatal neurologic or cardiac complications, such as prolonged seizures or disturbances of the heart rhythm.

Alleviation of Sleep Disorders

Sleep disturbances occasionally develop with multiple sclerosis and may lead to daytime fatigue. The individual does not rest adequately at night, so lost sleep must be made up during the day. What may actually be disturbed is the sleep-wake cycle that is a normal part of every person's daily activity rhythm. Excessive inactivity disrupts this cycle. A pattern of naps during the day leads to a need for sleep during the day and insomnia at night.

Medications, such as flurazepam (Dalmane) at a dose of 15 mg or clonazepam (Klonopin) at a dose of 0.5 mg each night, may restore the normal sleep-wake cycle, but the most important step toward restoring the cycle is adopting a rigid schedule of daily activity, with sleep minimized during the day. The time that the person goes to bed and the time for getting out of bed should be the same every day. The number of hours spent in bed should be limited to 6 to 9 hours, depending on the individual's customary needs. Someone who has always slept 7 hours a night will be restless and anxious if he or she stays in bed for 9 hours.

Managing Complications of Severe Disease

Several problems only develop in people who have severe disease for several years. The most common complications of severe disability include pressure sores on the skin, contractures of the limbs, and frequent urinary tract infections. Individuals with any of these problems are likely to have several of them because the level of disease required to cause any is severe enough to cause most.

Skin Care

Pressure over a small area of the skin for more than a few minutes can interfere with blood flow and threaten skin integrity. People normally shift their limbs and trunk every few minutes whenever they are sitting or lying down. If a limb is in a very awkward position, the individual will make a conscious effort to get into a more comfortable position, but most of the adjustments that are required to keep the body's surface uninjured are reflex actions. The reflex depends on the ability to sense pain or deep pressure and upon the ability to shift position, even if only by a few millimeters.

The person with severe multiple sclerosis may lose this reflex positioning because of problems in sensation or movement. If part of a limb does not sense pain, the affected person may leave it in a dangerous position for too long even if he or she is able to move the limb. A more common phenomenon in multiple sclerosis is that the person feels discomfort, but spasticity or weakness interferes with his or her ability to shift the position of the limb. The result is pressure sores. These sores, or *decubiti* (de-KYEW-bit-eye), may start as little more than blistering on the surface of the skin, but without proper attention can extend directly down to bone. They are easily infected and heal slowly even with the best management. Effective management often requires hospitalization.

In its early stages, the pressure sore or decubitus can be stopped by eliminating pressure from the affected area completely. Even when the skin appears damaged, efforts to keep it dry, free of debris, and out of contact with all hard surfaces may be enough to allow healing. Loose skin and deeper tissue that is no longer healthy must be cut away. Without this maneuver, which is called *debridement,* healing is slowed and infection progresses more quickly. Any skin infections that develop should be treated with antibiotics. The type of antibiotic used will be determined by the type of organism causing the infection.

If the individual developed the problem because of severe immobilization, a special surface may be required to prevent the worsening of pressure sores. Water beds are commonly used to reduce the amount of pressure on any one area of the skin. More sophisticated bed systems in which fine beads, rather than water, are circulated under an individual are available for managing the most severe cases, but in most situations they are not necessary.

An often-overlooked aspect of decubitus management is diet. Without adequate calories and vitamins, the battle against decubiti may be doomed to fail. Food supplements high in calories should be given to those who have poor nutrition because of decreased appetite or problems in eating. Vitamin supplements may be necessary, but should not be massive. A balanced diet with adequate calories, fats, vitamins, and proteins is preferable to supplements, but for some people, problems with eating or absorbing food make supplements necessary.

Because wet skin becomes injured more easily than dry skin, the patient must be kept dry as well as clean. Those with enough immobility to develop decubiti often have problems with bladder control; thus, incontinence complicates the management of the decubiti. A catheter left in the bladder may be needed as part of the decubitus care simply to keep skin surfaces dry.

With extensive loss of skin, healing may take too long to be practical. In such cases, plastic surgery becomes necessary to close the skin surface. Skin grafts used to cover the injured areas must themselves be protected against pressure injury. Without such precautions, the graft site does not heal and the graft fails.

In the severely impaired individual, decubiti should be looked for on a regular basis. Certain body surfaces, such as the base of the spine and the heels, are especially likely to develop pressure sores. These must be examined every day, and corrective measures must be started as soon as there is any evidence of skin breakdown. In all cases, the best management of decubiti is prevention, but for the severely impaired individual prevention may be impossible.

Therapy for Spasms and Spasticity

Spasticity may hold a limb in an unwanted position and thereby contribute to the development of decubiti. Although the skin problems associated with spasticity are the most dangerous of the common complications of profound spasticity, there are several other complications. With a limb held for a long time in one position, the person is likely to develop changes at the joints that themselves interfere with mobility, called *contractures*. With a contracture, the recovery of strength in a limb may be masked by the resistance to movement that develops as the limb freezes in the spastic position.

Involuntary contractions of spastic muscles are called *spasms.* These transient spasms may be severely painful and resistant to drugs that treat spasticity even if the underlying spasticity does respond. With such problems, the affected person may benefit from physical therapy that maintains the normal structure and mobility of the joints. A skilled therapist works to stretch any contracted tendons and relax muscles that frequently spasm. If joint deformity is allowed to develop as a result of the spasticity, the person will have more weakness and instability in the affected limb. More drastic measures are occasionally necessary when years of spasticity lead to virtually useless limbs that are a source of constant pain and recurrent decubiti. In such cases, surgical techniques may be used to relieve the spasticity.

Nerve Blocks

When paralysis has already been present for years and spasticity is producing intractable pain and skin damage, the individual may benefit from an irreversible block of the nerve. This does not necessarily require surgery. The injection of various toxic substances in or near the nerve may suffice to produce the irreversible damage.

Permanent interference with the operation of a nerve is a drastic step and should only be performed after all other options have been explored and the problem with spasticity has persisted long enough to establish that it will be permanent. Nerve blocks produced by the injection of toxic substances are usually performed by an experienced anesthesiologist or neurosurgeon. The possibility of injury to nerves that are not involved in the spasticity is too great to entrust this procedure to someone who has not performed it many times under supervision.

Where nerves travel closely together, surgery may be necessary to selectively block the nerve to the intended muscle. It is better to avoid surgery if possible, however, because people who are so severely impaired that a nerve block seems appropriate are usually not good surgical candidates. For instance, they may have pressure sores that will present problems during or after surgery.

If the same result can be achieved without damaging nerves, it is better to do that. With severe limb contractures, cutting the tendons may relieve pressure or pain, but this is much more substantial surgery than that required for cutting a nerve. It can only be done by an experienced orthopedic surgeon, and it requires a very sophisticated approach to the muscles, tendons, and joints.

Some neurosurgeons have attempted to manage spasticity in functionally useless limbs by making small incisions in the spinal cord. This is a dangerous technique in all but the most skilled neurosurgical hands and is rarely performed. The object of the surgery is to cut the fibers carrying the signal for contraction from upper motor nerve cells to lower motor nerve cells. This approach is no longer considered necessary or appropriate by most neurologists and neurosurgeons.

A related technique has involved the placement of electrical wires over the spinal cord. Because the electric contacts, or electrodes, are placed over the part of the spinal cord called the dorsal column, this technique is called *dorsal column stimulation*. It is generally not useful in the treatment of spasticity, but has found some application in the management of chronic pain. Very few neurosurgeons use dorsal column stimulation because its usefulness has not been proven.

Infection Control

Any condition that severely limits an individual's mobility will place him or her at risk for infection. Simply lying in bed increases the risk of pneumonia. As already mentioned, poor limb movements may produce decubiti that readily become infected. If superficial infections extend into the body tissues, they can produce abscesses or chronic bone infections. The most common site for infections in people with multiple sclerosis is the urinary tract. Regular elimination of urine either by drug-induced emptying of the bladder or by catheterization of the bladder reduces the risk of urinary tract infection but cannot eliminate it completely.

Physical therapy is an important part of the management of

infections. Keeping the person with multiple sclerosis active reduces the risk that infections will gain a foothold. An adequate diet is also important, but it is too often overlooked by those who rely on medication to suppress infections and who have a loss of appetite because of the chronic illness.

With recurrent bladder infections, the individual may need more or less chronic administration of antibiotics. As already mentioned above, Septra and Bactrim are two of the most commonly used preparations, and both are routinely used repeatedly because of the low risk that the infecting agents will develop resistance to the drugs.

With frequent bladder infections, kidney damage may develop; and with kidney damage, kidney failure may occur. Kidney failure is a life-threatening complication; aggressive measures must be taken to avoid this problem. In some cases the bladder becomes so nonfunctional that drainage from the kidneys must be rerouted to save the kidneys. Very few people with multiple sclerosis require this type of intervention, but it may be necessary for the severely impaired individual with intractable bladder and kidney infections.

CHAPTER 8

Social, Psychological, and Sexual Problems

The social and psychological costs of multiple sclerosis are enormous. The costs to society include the days of work missed, medical bills incurred, unemployment insurance paid, and social services required. These and other tangible expenses total more than $100 million a year in the United States alone. The psychological costs to the affected person, the family, and those dependent on the affected person are less easily expressed in dollars, but are no less substantial.

The social and psychological costs are greater with multiple sclerosis than with many other diseases simply because of the age at which it appears and does most of its damage. The affected individuals are in their childbearing and child-rearing years, at the beginning of job or career development, at an age when they are routinely expected to be independent. This disease affects all of these activities to some extent; the degree to which they are affected is determined as much by the personality and resources of the individual before the appearance of the demyelinating disease as by the deficits imposed by the disease.

Fear of Progressive Disability

With any chronic illness, the fear that the disease will cause progressive disability is unavoidable. With multiple sclerosis, this is especially true because some individuals with this disorder develop severe physical handicaps. What most people do not realize is that there are many people with multiple sclerosis who never develop significant handicaps. The poor outcomes of the disease are much more memorable and disturbing than the good outcomes, so apprehension is natural for people with multiple sclerosis.

This abiding fear can be disabling in itself. Young adults may be reluctant to marry, begin careers, or start families, because of the possible disruption threatened by progression of the disease. This behavior is especially likely if flare-ups of the disease have already interfered with the pursuit of a social or professional goal. Sexual difficulties may develop as a complication of the disease or as a reflection of psychological problems. Those problems directly arising from nervous system disease are often manageable; those related to psychological difficulties usually abate with professional help.

The fear of progressive disability and the emotional problems associated with multiple sclerosis are best dealt with by psychological counseling. Group discussions with other affected individuals often provide new viewpoints and alternative strategies. Self-help and counseling groups are usually more effective than individual therapy. National organizations, such as the National Multiple Sclerosis Society in the United States, sponsor and supervise such groups. These types of groups are useful for family members, as well as for the individual with multiple sclerosis, since they provide an outlet for much of the stress that disturbs the family of a person with this disease.

Employment Problems

Disabilities caused by multiple sclerosis may affect an individual's success at certain types of employment. For example, the high incidence of visual disorders may make tasks requiring good vision impractical. Both the affected person's abilities prior to developing symptoms and the disabilities acquired during the course of the illness will determine what types of employment are suitable.

Qualified people with multiple sclerosis usually do not encounter major barriers in employment if their specific talents or experience make them a real asset to the company, especially if they were regular employees before the disease appeared. Most people with mild or inapparent multiple sclerosis do not tell their employers that they have the disease since, in many cases, the initial episode and occasional flare-ups are mistaken for isolated illnesses. If severe flare-ups later make it impossible to conceal the disease, however, the employer may feel deceived.

Looking for a new job may be more difficult. The recent Americans with Disabilities Act, however, makes it illegal for most employers with at least 15 employees to discriminate against handicapped individuals in hiring, promotions, pay, fringe benefits, and other aspects of employment. A disabled person can only be legally excluded from a job if he or she is unable to perform the *essential* functions of the job. For instance, if the job description for a stock person says that the person must work in high places, but no one holding the job has had to work in high places for several years, that is not an essential function.

In addition, the law requires that employers must make "reasonable accommodations" for people with disabilities. This means that an employer may need to adjust the work environment to make the job safer for the disabled person, or may need to redistribute *nonessential* job functions to other employees. It is illegal for the employer to hire an individual who does not have a disability over an equally qualified disabled person in order to avoid making such reasonable accommodations. Of course, it is sometimes difficult to determine what type of accommodation is "reasonable." The applicant or employee should notify the employer about his or her needs, and then be willing to engage in a discussion of options. The Equal Employment Opportunity Commission (EEOC) or other agencies may be helpful.

Under the Americans with Disabilities Act, it is illegal on a job application or in an interview to ask questions specifically about whether a person has any medical disorders. It is permitted to ask whether the applicant can perform essential job functions and whether he or she will need any reasonable accommodation in the application process, such as more time to complete a written examination. The person applying may also be asked about the ability to perform nonessential functions in the job, but he or she cannot be denied employment solely because of problems with these marginal functions.

A prospective employer does have a right to know about an individual's prior work performance, so that if the person with multiple sclerosis has required an excessive amount of time off for flare-ups of the disease, he or she should try to show that such a pattern of absences will not be a problem in the future, or, if it may continue to be a problem, that he or she will be an asset to the company anyway because of talents and experience. Specialized vocational training may help the individual to compete more effectively in this way.

Obviously, disclosing the disease eliminates a source of stress in employment. When instability in walking or slurred speech develops at work, it is better to be recognized as a person with multiple sclerosis than to be thought drugged or intoxicated. How the disclosure is made is very important, however. Because most people know little about the disease, what is said should be carefully planned to inform but not terrify the employer or co-workers. The individual with multiple sclerosis should discuss what to say with a physician familiar with his or her circumstances and then rehearse the presentation. The disclosure should be made in a calm, organized way, avoiding medical jargon, and the affected individual must be ready to answer questions about the illness. The individual must appear comfortable with his or her own skills and disabilities. In general, one should be specific in describing the actual limitations imposed by the disease, but emphasize abilities, not disabilities. A letter from a physician supporting the specifics of the disclosure may reassure a wary employer.

Family Adjustment

Relatives of the person with multiple sclerosis usually have many concerns brought on by their perception of the disease. Many worry that they, too, might be susceptible to multiple sclerosis because of hereditary factors. More reasonable concerns include changes in the role that will be played by the afflicted family member if the neurologic disease progresses. The role played by a woman with several children who has minor visual problems is very different from that played by the same woman if she develops significant leg weakness. Both the nature of the family and the nature of the neurologic signs and symptoms will determine the adjustments that must be made by the family members.

Promoting Independence

What the family must do to adjust to the multiple sclerosis has many aspects. Disabilities must not be exaggerated. It is natural to encourage someone with an illness to become less active and less independent throughout the illness, but this is neither reasonable nor desirable in a condition such as multiple sclerosis that may be active for many years and leave neurologic problems that persist for life. Neither activity nor stress should be eliminated from the individual's life. Especially when the person with the disease is relatively young, the family is likely to shelter the individual from all types of stress. Self-sufficiency is often discouraged, a practice that works against the person's maximizing his or her independence.

Eliminating Guilt and Accusations

In many families, the true nature of the problem is distorted. At worst, the family members see the disease as a judgment from a divine source on the person with multiple sclerosis or on the family as a whole. "What did we do to deserve this?" often becomes much more than a rhetorical question. Accusations growing out of this sense of guilt can easily fragment a family.

Several characteristics of multiple sclerosis have an especially erosive influence on the family. If the affected individual has relatively subtle signs and symptoms, such as poor vision and easy fatigability, but can no longer make a significant contribution to the family, the subtlety of the problem may arouse considerable animosity. The impaired individual may be seen by other members of the family as exploiting the neurologic problem. Even when family members do not suggest that the person is not helping out, an overly sensitive individual may feel constantly obliged to prove that he or she really is not healthy. This may provoke activities that worsen the condition and place additional strains on the family.

Redistributing Responsibilities

When someone has been an active and contributing member of the family, it is often devastating to discover suddenly that routine activities cannot be consistently performed. The young mother may find that she simply does not have the energy to manage her children every day. Establishing consistent patterns of exertion and pacing herself may help much of the time, but the family as a group must devise strategies for picking up the slack when she cannot do the most routine activities. Devising such an alternative strategy is truly the responsibility of the entire family. The person with the neurologic disease should not be obliged to assign responsibilities to other family members. Professional counseling is usually needed to devise these strategies.

Distributing Resources

Also destructive to the family's working as a unit for the benefit of all its members is the dedication of a disproportionate a part of the resources of the family to the person with multiple sclerosis. When the disease is especially active or the nervous system destruction is especially severe, most of the family's resources and attention may be needed to support the affected person, but when that extraordinary diversion of resources is no longer essential, it should no longer be provided. The children of a parent with multiple sclerosis suffer unduly when one spouse dedicates all available time and energy to the care of the other. When the individual with multiple sclerosis needs a great deal of attention, it should be available, but when not essential, it should be distributed in a more equitable manner.

Venting Emotions

The disability and dependence imposed by the nervous system disease often inhibits the ability of the person with multiple sclerosis to vent emotions. It is awkward to express anger at the people to whom one is indebted for all types of assistance, but this type of expression is important in every family. When anger cannot be outwardly expressed, it is focused inward, and generally manifests itself as depression. What family members must understand is that much of the bitterness and anger felt by the person with multiple sclerosis is directed at them simply because they are there. Anger must have a target, and the nearest person usually becomes that target. That family members are not appropriate objects of this ill-feeling usually becomes obvious to both the individual with multiple sclerosis and the family after the anger has been allowed to surface. Family encounter groups under the supervision of an experienced psychologist or family therapist generally provide the best arena in which this anger can surface and be defused.

Depression and Emotional Instability

Depression is a common problem with any chronic illness. In multiple sclerosis, as opposed to most other long-term health problems, depression may be a reaction to the disease, a consequence of the disease, or a side effect of treatment (Table 8–1). Damage to the nervous system can cause mood disturbances, and severe depression may be a sign of severe disease. Mood changes may flare up, just as visual problems, weakness, and bladder disturbances can develop with exacerbations of the disease. This is not to say that individuals necessarily become depressed with worsening of their condition. During a flare-up, the person with multiple sclerosis may show no personality or mood changes or may even become inappropriately euphoric.

**TABLE 8–1. Some Causes of Depression
in MS**

Stress
Demyelination
Steroid withdrawal
Drug reaction

Which mood changes, if any, will occur is unpredictable. Depression is the most problematic of the mood disturbances because it is the most disabling. The depressed person loses interest in social activities and may become self-destructive. Loss of weight, problems with sleeping, and withdrawal from family and friends often signal the development of a severe depression. Regardless of whether or not the depression can be tied to a flare-up of the multiple sclerosis, it must be treated with all the care appropriate for any episode of serious depression. Professional help is needed in this situation. An understanding family is important, but not sufficient.

Drug-related Depression

Some of the drugs used in the management of multiple sclerosis cause depression. Rare individuals taking high doses of steroids will have agitation and destructive behavior that lessen as the dosage of steroids is tapered. Mood changes are especially common when the person is being treated with corticosteroids, such as prednisone, cortisone acetate, dexamethasone (Decadron), and methylprednisolone. Whenever a person's dosage of steroids is reduced, depression may appear. This should be anticipated and minimized as much as possible. The best way to reduce the severity of the depression is to taper the steroid dosage gradually.

If severe depression develops despite a gradual reduction in the dosage of the steroids, antidepressant medication may be appropriate. A neurologist or psychiatrist familiar with the psychological complications of multiple sclerosis should decide which type of treatment is appropriate.

Drugs meant to reduce the frequency of flare-ups, such as interferon beta-1b (Betaseron), or the complications of multiple sclerosis, such as oxybutinin (Ditropan) for bladder disturbances and methocarbamol (Robaxin) for muscle pain, may also cause mood disturbances. Whenever severe depression appears with the introduction of a new medication, it is reasonable to stop the medication. If the depression clears as the medication is eliminated from the body, the drug should be avoided in the future.

Treatment of Depression with Drugs

The depression that appears in many people with multiple sclerosis is as treatable as the depression that appears with other types of nervous system disease. This depression responds to a variety of medications. Psychotherapy may be helpful over the course of years, but for the depression that more clearly appears as part of a flare-up or as one of the effects of several nervous system injuries, antidepressant drug should suffice. Fluoxetine (Prozac), imipramine (Tofranil), and amitriptyline (Elavil) are widely prescribed and are usually safe and effective for people with depression and multiple sclerosis.

Fluoxetine has gained considerable popularity in recent years because it is an antidepressant with a relatively benign side-effect profile. It can be taken orally as a single dose of 20 mg daily.

Imipramine is generally taken in a single dose of 100 to 150 mg at bedtime. It must be taken regularly, whether or not the person feels especially depressed on any particular day. Drowsiness develops in many people within a few hours after the dose, so it is best taken just before going to sleep.

Amitriptyline is closely related to imipramine chemically, but some people have fewer side effects and notice much less drowsiness. This drug can be taken in small doses during the day, such as 10 to 25 mg two to three times daily. Both imipramine and amitriptyline usually cause dryness in the mouth and a metallic taste and may cause problems with bladder control. They interfere slightly with bladder emptying and may produce substantial urinary retention if the individual already has mild bladder problems.

Central nervous system complications, such as disturbed thinking, abnormal body temperatures, or altered blood pressure control, must be watched for in those people who are taking any of these antidepressant drugs because of the already disturbed function of their nervous system. Women should avoid pregnancy or breast-feeding while taking these drugs, to avoid injury to the fetus or infant. Electroshock therapy is not appropriate as part of the management of the depression unless the individual has a psychotic emotional disorder unrelated to the multiple sclerosis.

Follow-up for Depression

The depressed person with multiple sclerosis must be watched as carefully as any depressed individual because of the risk of self-destructive behavior. If there is any risk of suicide, the affected person should be hospitalized. The depression will respond to treatment and the person will again function safely at home, but a physician familiar with depression in its various forms should decide when it is safe for the affected individual to be at home alone; this decision cannot be left to the individual or the family. It is often the person whose depression seems to lift abruptly who has finally formulated and decided to act on a plan for suicide.

Disturbances of Sexual Activity

Most people with multiple sclerosis are sexually active when they develop their first symptoms of disease. The appearance of multiple sclerosis has a substantial impact on that sexual activity, but the impact usually is not the result of disturbed nervous-system control of sexual organs. Indeed, much of the disturbance in sexual activity occurs because the person with multiple sclerosis is concerned about the way he or she is viewed by his or her sexual partner. Compounding the problem are the concerns of the individual's sexual partner, who may worry that sex is painful or burdensome for the person with neurologic disease.

With any chronic illness, the frequency or character of sexual activity usually changes. Even though multiple sclerosis is characterized by periods of improvement and worsening, sexual activity may be affected during intervals when the person has no symptoms of active disease. For many, the impact of multiple sclerosis on self-image causes the change in sexual activity. For others, the persistent disability associated with repeated attacks of the illness disturbs sexual patterns.

Sexual activity serves many functions, ranging from relaxation to reproduction. Which of these functions is most important for the individual will affect what adjustments must be made in sexual activity. The sexual problems imposed by multiple sclerosis range from bouts of fatigue that interfere with protracted intercourse to loss of the ability to have intercourse. Changes in sensation in the penis or vagina are certainly much more common than impotence or unreceptiveness. This sensory disturbance may produce little sensation or painful sensations with attempts at intercourse. Even when this fundamental part of sexual activity is impaired, it is important to remember that a great deal of sexual satisfaction is possible without successful or even attempted intercourse.

Exertion and Contraception

Sexual dilemmas facing men and women with multiple sclerosis are, of course, as different as their sexual interests. Men are often concerned about the effect of frequent sexual exertion on the course of their illness, whereas women more often worry about the effect of various contraceptive methods on their disease. In fact, sexual activity should not worsen (or improve) the course of multiple sclerosis for either men or women. As with any physical activity, extreme exhaustion should be avoided by people with multiple sclerosis. Men routinely feel somewhat sedated after sexual climax, but this apparent fatigue should not be misconstrued as exhaustion. A concerned sexual partner who limits sexual activity in an effort to conserve the affected individual's strength may do no good for the nervous system disease, but will usually undermine the sexual relationship with this strategy.

Women can use any of the currently popular birth control measures with no reservations. Birth control pills do not cause an increased incidence of relapses. The mechanical devices currently and recently available, such as intrauterine devices (IUDs), diaphragms, sponges, and cervical caps, are practical if the women does not have a substantial problem with spasticity. Abdominal spasms do not increase the normally very small risk of uterine perforation with an IUD, but they may greatly increase the women's discomfort.

Sexual Problems Unrelated to Multiple Sclerosis

Sexual function is normal in most young people with multiple sclerosis. Problems with impotence, pain on intercourse, poor vaginal lubrication, impaired ejaculation, or sexual disinterest should be investigated for possible causes other than the multiple sclerosis. Common diseases such as diabetes mellitus and venereal infections can cause sexual problems in both men and women. Hormones essential for normal sexual activity are not affected by multiple sclerosis, and any disturbances in these substances must be explained by another mechanism.

Sexual Problems Caused by Multiple Sclerosis

Although sexual problems are not invariably present with multiple sclerosis, sexual function can be impaired on the basis of the multiple sclerosis alone. The difficulties may be strictly mechanical. A woman with spasticity in her legs may find it difficult or impossible to position herself to receive a sexual partner. This is much less likely than that problems with vaginal lubrication or relaxation of the muscles near the vagina may interfere with intercourse. Her partner may find attempts at penetration simply too painful for him to try.

For men with multiple sclerosis, sexual limitations may be more obvious. **Impotence** (that is, the inability to achieve or sustain an erection of the penis) may make sexual intercourse impossible. Even when the man can have an erection, orgasm may be painful because of poor coordination of the muscles involved in forcing the sperm along the delivery system from the testicles to the penis. Orgasm in men consists of several phases. The phase in which semen is driven out of the penis is called *ejaculation.* If muscle coordination is faulty, ejaculation may occur much sooner than the man wishes or intends, in which case it is called *premature ejaculation,* or it may direct the semen backward and result in a **retrograde ejaculation.**

Delayed, absent, or premature ejaculations are the most common sexual complaints of men with multiple sclerosis. Retrograde ejaculation may be so uncomfortable that the man with multiple sclerosis quickly learns to avoid sexual activity. Some men and women, discovering that they simply cannot achieve orgasm, are discouraged by this disability, and become sexually inactive.

About 25 to 40 percent of men between 18 and 50 years of age with multiple sclerosis are unable to have an erection or are unable to sustain an erection long enough during sexual intercourse to satisfy their partners. Even though the person with multiple sclerosis may have enough sexual ability intact to satisfy his own desires, the failure to satisfy his mate may undermine an important relationship. This sexual disability may be substantial even when little or no nervous system damage is apparent.

Women also have problems with several aspects of sexual activity, including achieving orgasm. Sexual problems affect more than half the sexually active women who have multiple sclerosis. As many as 36 percent of women have problems with vaginal lubrication, and 12 percent have discomfort when their genitals are fondled.

A woman's ability to have an orgasm is not necessarily lost with central nervous system damage. In fact, even with extensive nervous system impairment and complete loss of genital sensation, orgasm may still occur. What causes problems for women with multiple sclerosis is usually a combination of factors. A major factor is poor vaginal lubrication. What is usually erotic stimulation may produce unpleasant or painful sensations if vaginal lubrication is poor. Even if problems with sensation or lubrication do not occur, the woman with multiple sclerosis may experience pelvic muscle spasms during intercourse that cause considerable pain for her and frustrate her partner's efforts to penetrate the vaginal opening.

Emotional Components

With any sexual problem, there is a tendency to overestimate the emotional component of the problem. The sexual dysfunctions that develop in both men and women with demyelinating disease are usually physical disturbances more closely tied to spinal cord or brain disease than to fatigue or anxiety. The emotional impact of sexual dysfunction is, however, great and cannot be ignored. Most couples communicate poorly when it comes to sexual matters, and so a difficult sexual problem is often worsened by misinterpretations and feelings of rejection.

Management of Sexual Problems

No amount of disability imposed by multiple sclerosis should eliminate the affected person's sex life. Adjustments in sexual behavior may be necessary, but most people with this problem retain sexual interest and sexual needs. Sexual partners may have to make substantial changes in the types of activities in which they engage, but whatever is acceptable and enjoyable for the people involved should be explored. The first step in any sexual adjustment is trying to decide what changes have taken place in the individual's sex life and which of these changes are important for the affected person. Once the important problems have been identified, strategies for rebuilding or modifying sexual activity to make it more satisfying can be devised.

The first step requires an unusual degree of frankness. Simply to clarify the problems that have developed because of the multiple sclerosis, most couples will need someone to help them explore these highly sensitive areas. An experienced sex therapist is usually best qualified to serve as this intermediary. Involving other couples with similar problems is also a very effective and acceptable way of discussing sexual problems. A group discussion of sexual limitations is generally much less inhibiting than a discussion just between the two sexual partners. Once the problems have been identified, they may be overcome.

Alternatives to Intercourse

Obviously, there is much more to sexual activity than sexual intercourse, and what is of interest to both sexual partners should be pursued. Genital stimulation may bring a man or a woman to orgasm even when vaginal penetration or penile erection are impossible. Individuals with limited mobility may find oral sex is a more practical alternative than strictly manual stimulation. Use of vibrators or other materials to improve sexual arousal may allow the couple to engage in a great deal of sexual activity while using little energy.

If vaginal penetration is important for the couple and the man cannot achieve a satisfactory erection, the partners may find simple manual techniques effective. The woman can manipulate the non-erect penis to get it into her vagina. With constriction of her pelvic muscles around the vagina, some enlargement of the penis may occur; even if it does not, the vaginal contact may be satisfying for both partners.

Penile Implants and Injections

Penile implants may assist sexually impaired men in achieving erections, but the surgery is delicate and the results are quite inconsistent. These implants do not provide an alternative to poor erections and are not appropriate for men who still can muster enough firmness in the penis to allow intercourse. Implants are usually performed by urologists (physicians who treat the urinary tract and male genitals) with special experience in this area.

A simpler and more reliable technique involves the injection into the penis of drugs that induce an erection. Which drugs can be used and which procedure should be followed must be determined by an experienced urologist. Drugs commonly used include prostaglandin E_1, phentolamine, and papaverine. These drugs work by activating vascular reflexes that have been disconnected from spinal cord pathways in some individuals with multiple sclerosis. Without attention to appropriate dosing and technique, however, the patient may injure the penis by causing a very prolonged erection (priapism) or scar tissue.

Spasticity and Sexual Activity

Spasms of the muscles on the inner aspects of the thighs may interfere with sexual intercourse whether the affected individual is male or female. Antispasticity agents may be helpful, or changes in position may be necessary. What bars vaginal entry from the front may not cause problems when the man attempts entry from the back. If there is poor vaginal lubrication, the affected woman can use an artificial lubricant. Applying this material can become a part of foreplay without disrupting the couple's usual sexual pattern.

Sex and Incontinence

Problems with reflexes controlled by the lower spinal cord are usually responsible for lapses in voluntary control of the bladder or bowels. Because this same area of the spinal cord is important in normal sexual function, it is common for individuals to have both sexual problems and incontinence. Avoiding bladder or bowel incontinence during sexual activity may require a trip to the bathroom before sexual encounters, but the security provided by this routine usually justifies the inconvenience imposed on sexual partners. Restricting fluid intake prior to expected sexual activity may also reduce the probability of an accident during intercourse or genital stimulation. Eating increases intestinal activity, and so sexual encounters are better before a meal than after it.

   Pressure on the bladder is enough in some cases to produce urinary incontinence. If the affected individual finds that even with emptying his or her bladder before intercourse, bladder pressure still produces some dribbling, then different positions should be attempted. If the affected partner is a woman, less pressure will be exerted on the bladder if her partner does not lie on top of her abdomen. Entry would be less stressful if her partner mounted her from the back or if she sat on him as he lay on his back. Other variations in position that minimize pressure on the lower abdomen can be devised with experimentation.

Individuals with in-dwelling bladder catheters may still be sexually active, but removal and reinsertion of the catheter before and after sexual intercourse may be impractical. Women with catheters may fasten them out of the way by taping them to the front of the groin. Men with catheters may need to fold the tube back over the penis and secure it with a condom drawn over both the penis and the tube.

Bladder infections are a routine concern for individuals with poor bladder control, and this is worsened if the affected person has both poor bladder and poor bowel control. Bathing at the time of sexual encounters may be both sexually stimulating and reassuring to the individual who has problems with recurrent bladder infections triggered by sexual activity.

Psychological Adjustments

Attempts at improving sexual satisfaction should not take on the character of a holy crusade. The wife who works to bring her husband to orgasm and feels frustration and anger when all her attention fails is doing little except cooling her husband's interest in trying to have sexual intercourse. The husband who makes no sexual overtures to his wife because she may develop painful vaginal spasms on attempts at penetration is simply eliminating sex from the relationship. For those couples who are exploring new sexual techniques, it often does more harm than good to constantly quiz each other on what feels good. Discussions when the couple is not engaged in sexual activity or comments about what does not feel good during sexual contacts may be enough to ensure that both parties are satisfied. All such discussions are most fruitful if they are directed by a therapist familiar with the sexual problems resulting from multiple sclerosis.

Developing Sexual Relationships

For many people, multiple sclerosis appears before they have acquired much or any sexual experience. This imposes the additional problem of developing competence in sexuality at the same time that physical problems may limit sexual performance. Meeting people and developing intimate relationships is always difficult but it may be especially problematic when problems with walking, bladder control, or even vision limit the individual's spontaneity and independence. This does not mean that people with symptoms of multiple sclerosis cannot develop very rich sex lives. It simply means that there may be special barriers requiring special approaches.

For unimpaired individuals, intimacy usually starts as a non-sexual relationship, and so it must be for people with physical disabilities. Frankness can help disarm many of the apprehensions unavoidable in the relationship between a person with multiple sclerosis and a potential lover. The disabled person is wise to be explicit in asking for any necessary assistance, but should be careful not to be manipulative. The more that is revealed, the fewer the misconceptions and fears that can develop between the two people involved in the relationship. In any evolving friendship, there is the potential for a sexual relationship, and so the most direct route to a sexual relationship is through a friendship. People with similar interests and activities should be sought out.

Self-stimulation

Self-stimulation by masturbation or other erotic activities may help the person with multiple sclerosis to relax, as well as to find out what type of stimulation is most satisfying. This self-awareness is especially important when a sexual relationship begins and the partners experiment with different types of sexual activity. Knowing what is comfortable and what is unpleasant helps the partners to achieve the most satisfaction that they can experience early in the sexual relationship. Men may find that touching certain parts of the penis produces no sensation or pain. Women may find that mechanical aids such as vibrators and dildos provide more stimulation than intercourse or massage. Whatever technique is most satisfying should become familiar to the person with multiple sclerosis through experimentation. The person with multiple sclerosis, like the person with no nervous system disease, has the best chance of developing satisfying sexual relationships if he or she is already comfortable with his or her own sexuality and sexual interests.

Homosexuality

In the general population of the United States, about 1 to 2 percent of individuals prefer to have or strive to have exclusively homosexual sexual relations. People with multiple sclerosis are neither more nor less likely to be heterosexual than the rest of the population. There certainly are homosexual people with this nervous system disease, and their sexual concerns are as substantial as for those who are heterosexual. In many cities, the homosexual community is more closely knit than the heterosexual community, and this camaraderie can be a valuable asset to the person with disabilities that might interfere with the evolution of sexual relationships.

Aphrodisiacs

There are no drugs or vitamins that will predictably improve sexual performance or heighten sexual interest. Many people claim that a certain hormone or vitamin results in spectacular changes in their sexual activity, but these aphrodisiac effects are generally false or limited to a few individuals. The person may experience a placebo effect that has a dramatic impact on performance, but by definition this effect is mediated by the person's expectations rather than by any property of the drug.

Vitamin E is one of the commonly advertised aphrodisiacs, despite clear evidence that it has no measurable effect on sexual interest or activity. Sex hormones, such as the male hormone testosterone, do affect sexual interest in both men and women when they are produced by the individual's own glands. Testosterone pills or elixirs are not effective, and injections are more likely simply to depress one's own hormone production than to substantially affect sexual behavior. There are risks associated with taking any unneeded hormone, and the person with multiple sclerosis should not be exposed to them simply on the outside chance that a placebo effect might occur.

Cocaine and other illicit drugs have been touted as aphrodisiacs, but any change in sexual activity observed with these substances is difficult to assess because of the lack of controlled, scientific studies. The sense of well-being and competence that many people report while taking cocaine may lead to changes in sexual activity as part of a widespread neurologic alteration. That all the neurologic changes occurring are harmless is unlikely in the person without multiple sclerosis and inconceivable in the person with multiple sclerosis. Some of the commonly abused drugs, such as barbiturates, depress central nervous system activity; they cannot improve sexual performance, but may substantially impair it.

Effects of MS Therapy

The treatment of nonsexual complications of multiple sclerosis may cause sexual problems. If a man is taking a tranquilizing drug to manage a disease-related mood disorder, that drug may interfere with erection and ejaculation. Tranquilizing drugs, as well as drugs to lessen spasticity, may also lessen a man's or a woman's sexual interest. If antidepressants are used, they may interfere with erection for the man and with vaginal lubrication and clitoral engorgement for the woman. It is important that people with multiple sclerosis be aware that these treatments can affect their sexual activity so that they do not assume that they have yet another problem. The drugs causing the problem need not be stopped, but changes in dosage or drug type may reduce the unwanted side effects.

Birth Control

Multiple sclerosis does not reduce an individual's fertility. As with any illness, severe disability may alter factors important in reproduction and make conception more difficult, but most people with multiple sclerosis must consider themselves as likely to cause or have a pregnancy as unaffected individuals. This means that couples not interested in reproducing must use birth control devices or drugs or submit to sterilization. The technique most suited to the couple should be determined partly by which partner is affected by the demyelinating disease and partly by what type of problems the affected individual has as a result of the multiple sclerosis.

With mild disease, all the contraceptive devices and techniques available to unaffected individuals are useful and appropriate for those with multiple sclerosis. With more severe disease, some of these become impractical. If the affected woman has spasms in the thighs that interfere with separating the legs, placement of a diaphragm before intercourse becomes impractical. Men who have poor erections can still make their partners pregnant if they take no contraceptive measures, but their problems with developing or maintaining an erection may interfere with retaining a condom on the penis. In many cases, the affected woman or man may have to rely heavily on contraceptive precautions taken by the unaffected sexual partner.

If problems with menstrual hygiene arise, the woman with multiple sclerosis is wise to avoid IUDs. When menstruation is obstructed by abnormal muscle activity in the thighs or groin, the risk of pelvic infections that accompanies the use of these devices is slightly increased. Such infections may go undetected for days or weeks, during which time the woman appears to have a flare-up of the multiple sclerosis.

Sterilization is a safe and reasonable option for individuals who have all the children they want. A vasectomy or tubal ligation can be done with local anesthesia and virtually no convalescence. This is generally an irreversible measure and is appropriate only when the person undergoing it is under no undue pressure to submit to the procedure.

Pregnancy

Pregnancy is probably not a cause of additional problems for the woman with multiple sclerosis, but child rearing may be impractical for severely disabled women. There is no clear evidence of increased relapses during an uncomplicated pregnancy, but some investigators have found a 20 percent risk of exacerbation during the first few weeks or months after the delivery. Regardless of the short-term effects of the pregnancy, it is clear that the long-term outcome for the affected woman is no poorer if she has a child or does not.

Most women who become pregnant are in their teens or twenties, and this is precisely the time when the demyelinating disease usually first appears. What is not obvious to the 19-year-old woman is whether or not she will be able to care for a child when she is 24 years old. If she has had only one or two flare-ups at the time she gets pregnant, chances are good that she will have little or no real disability as she enters motherhood. Unfortunately, the true severity of the disease is usually not obvious until the patient has had the disease for at least 5 years. The minimally impaired woman who gets pregnant at 19 years of age may be an extremely dependent and relatively immobile individual when she is 24 years of age. For some women, this will not affect the decision to have children, but it is a consideration that both parents must face.

Rather than deciding whether or not to have a family when the disease is first diagnosed, it is usually more reasonable to wait. What will become obvious over the course of a few years is whether or not the woman with multiple sclerosis is likely to be severely limited in her activities by the disease and, if incapacity develops, whether or not it is practical for the couple to rear a child. Many women in wheelchairs decide they want to have children, but the full implications of immobility and dependence are difficult for anyone to appreciate when they have not experienced the problem.

For most women, the wait of 3, 4, or even 5 years will still place them well within the years most practical for childbearing. For most women with multiple sclerosis, child rearing will be practical even if a few episodes of demyelination have occurred. The person who must critically assess her motives and abilities is the woman who has developed substantial disabilities early in the course of the illness. In many cases, motherhood is sought by these severely impaired women in an ill-fated effort to secure some happiness in the face of illness, but the demands of children may be much more than the severely affected woman can manage. A strenuous effort to provide what a normal child wants and needs may exhaust the mother with multiple sclerosis and interfere with her rearing of the child. If the parents have substantial financial or family resources, the rearing of a child may demand little physical exertion by the mother and becomes a much less complex decision for both parents.

If a woman with MS wants to have children, there is usually no reason why she cannot attempt to have a child, unless there are enormous physical complications of the nervous system disease. The nervous system disease does not cause insurmountable problems with fertility, and once conception has occurred, the pregnancy will not worsen the demyelinating disease. Of course, for men with multiple sclerosis, their concerns with reproduction are not the adverse effects of pregnancy, but rather problems with fertility and child rearing.

Barriers to Pregnancy

Women with spastic contractures of the legs or spasticity in the muscles about the vagina may find that sexual intercourse is not a practical route to becoming pregnant. Fortunately there are alternative routes. Artificial insemination has reached the level of routine procedure in most medical centers and fertility clinics. This procedure involves the introduction of semen into the vagina by strictly mechanical methods. The woman's mate provides the semen in most circumstances. All he need do is masturbate to produce the sample. If that is not practical, a sperm bank can provide the sample for insemination.

In some cases, the barrier to pregnancy is that multiple sclerosis affects the man, not the woman. If a man has disease affecting his spinal cord reflex, ejaculation may be defective and impregnation of his mate by conventional sexual encounters may be impractical. An alternative to intercourse is pooling of semen collected from the affected man. This semen can be used for artificial insemination. In some men, spinal cord injuries alter the content of the semen, rather than interfere with ejaculation. The level of sperm in the semen must be adequate to allow conception before impregnation becomes possible. If necessary the semen can be artificially manipulated to increase the sperm concentration, and then used in artificial insemination. If this is not effective, the couple must consider other alternatives if they are still committed to having a child. Use of sperm from a donor or adoption of a child may be the only available options.

Impact on Multiple Sclerosis

Pregnancy has no significant ill effects on the immediate or later course of multiple sclerosis. That the nervous system disease may complicate impregnation, labor and delivery, and child rearing is undeniable, but there is no good evidence that childbearing will worsen the nervous system disease. There is some evidence, in fact, that flare-ups of multiple sclerosis are less likely when a woman with the disease is pregnant. Some women do have the first symptom of multiple sclerosis during a pregnancy, but those women exhibit milder courses than women with disease first appearing when they are not pregnant.

The basis for this protective effect of pregnancy is presumed to involve a hormone or hormones that act on the immune system. During pregnancy, the immune system tolerates the presence of the fetus, which is immunologically a foreign body. Ordinarily, the immune system mounts a massive reaction to foreign bodies, and so the easing of immune reactions to allow development of the fetus may be instrumental in limiting attacks on the nervous system that are part of the demyelinating process.

This does not mean that very active multiple sclerosis will improve if the woman becomes pregnant. A woman with very active disease may find pregnancy an additional burden that she simply cannot tolerate. The pregnancy should be attempted during an interval when disease is not extremely active.

After the child is born, the mother is actually at an increased risk of a flare-up. The highest-risk period is during the first 6 to 9 months after the delivery. One out of five women with multiple sclerosis will have some signs of a flare-up during this period. Problems need not occur, but the parents should be prepared to obtain help to care for the child if there is a flare-up.

Delivery

The delivery is usually not complicated for the woman with multiple sclerosis. Adjustments must be made for the nervous system disease, but this only means that an experienced obstetrician and anesthesiologist, aware of the history of nervous system disease, should be involved in the delivery. Delivery by a midwife or other paramedical individual is unwise. If anesthetics or muscle relaxants are used, the amount must be modified to adjust for the nervous system sensitivity to such agents. Some physicians recommend avoiding spinal anesthetics because of the risk of worsening the multiple sclerosis.

If spasticity interferes with relaxation of muscles in the pelvis, a cesarean section may be necessary. In fact, few affected women need cesarean sections. The spasticity is rarely substantial in the vaginal region in women who decide to have children. These women tend to be under 25 years of age and to have minimal disability as result of the multiple sclerosis.

Breast-feeding

There is no danger of transferring multiple sclerosis to the baby through breast-feeding. Whether the mother can withstand the nutritional drain involved in breast-feeding a baby is a question to be decided by her and her gynecologist, but for most women with multiple sclerosis it is feasible. Part of the early care and feeding of the infant involves keeping an irregular schedule, and this may be deleterious to the mother's health. As already mentioned, the risk of flare-ups is greatest during the first 6 to 9 months after delivery, and it is during this time that the mother will be most fatigued if she tries to feed the baby at all hours of day and night. The satisfaction of rearing and caring for the infant must be balanced against the fatigue that develops with these activities. Whenever possible, the woman with multiple sclerosis should accept assistance in caring for her infant.

Child Rearing

Any person who decides to have children must consider the long-term consequences of this decision. If it is a man with multiple sclerosis, then his mate must decide on the pregnancy with a clear understanding of what her partner may be capable of contributing to the child's care and instruction over the course of years. If it is the woman who has the disease, she must recognize the problems that may lie ahead for both her and the child as the multiple sclerosis follows its course. These considerations will stop very few people from having children, but the pleasures of child rearing should be balanced against the burdens that it imposes.

CHAPTER 9

Lifestyle Adjustments

Lifestyle adjustments are unnecessary if the person with multiple sclerosis has no significant disabilities. Any changes in habits, clothing, shelter, or transportation that must be adopted are strictly determined by the problems caused by the disease. There are no changes in lifestyle that can protect the individual from progression of the disease or place him or her at additional risk of progressive disability. Attention to health is, of course, appropriate, but measures to avoid exhaustion, dehydration, overexposure, and malnutrition are as important for anyone else as they are for the person with multiple sclerosis. What is different for the person with demyelinating disease is the consequence of ignoring routine needs and reasonable precautions. A person without neurologic disease may feel exhausted with dehydration, but the person with multiple sclerosis and dehydration is likely to develop transient neurologic problems. Physical stress may revive deficits apparent during flare-ups months or years earlier.

If the individual with multiple sclerosis develops disabilities that interfere with normal activity, those limitations must be recognized, assessed, and managed. It is neither appropriate nor

161

helpful to ignore the problems imposed by the disease. Such denial can only compound the difficulties faced. Alternatively, it is a mistake to overrate the problems faced by an individual and limit that individual's independence because of an unrealistic assessment.

Visual Problems

The most common visual problems experienced by people with multiple sclerosis are blurred vision, double vision, and the illusion of movement. Blurred vision results from loss of visual acuity (that is, sharpness). Damage to the optic nerve does not affect the clarity of the image reaching the light receptors in the eye, but it does reduce the amount of information that is accurately transferred from the eye to the brain. Problems in the brain or at the base of the brain, in the brain stem, can interfere with the coordination of eye movements and produce either split images or the illusion of movement.

Blurred Vision

Because damage to the optic nerve is one of the most common complications of multiple sclerosis, many individuals with this disease must make changes in their habits and activities to compensate for poor vision. Problems with visual acuity may be somewhat helped by glasses or contact lenses, but the restoration of vision to normal is unlikely and this visual disability must be translated into changes, and in some cases restrictions, in activity. Driving may become dangerous if acuity drops sufficiently. Reading may become exhausting.

Alternative transportation must be found if operating a motor vehicle is too demanding a task. What the visually impaired person must determine is whether both acuity and field of vision are good enough to permit driving under any circumstances that might arise. It is unreasonable and negligent to drive when vision is only adequate with full illumination of all objects on and about the road. Daylight cannot be counted on even in regions with little rainfall. The eyes must be able to make abrupt adjustments in a wide range of light situations. The National Multiple Sclerosis Society in the United States can advise the person who needs help with transportation as to what resources are available in his or her region.

If reading is difficult, a variety of visual aids designed for people with severe visual impairments are available. Oversized type is the simplest adjustment, but books and papers printed with these large letters are relatively limited. Magnifying devices are more readily available and suffices for most people with the types of visual changes likely with multiple sclerosis. For the most severely impaired, recordings of books and braille transcriptions may be the only practical way to review printed material. The American Printing House and the Library of Congress provide books and other types of written material in large print and as recordings.

Some people with multiple sclerosis find that tinted lenses help their acuity by reducing glare. In the environment that the visually impaired person can control directly, increasing the contrast between items will reduce the risk of accidents. In the home, for instance, thresholds, exposed pipes, steps, and other items requiring some degree of attention to navigate around can be marked off in high-contrast paints. Those individuals who have lost color perception must use the acuity they have left to identify patterns that are as revealing as colors. Remembering that the stop light is at the top of the traffic signal column becomes an essential part of driving.

Double Vision

Problems with eye movements can interfere with vision. If coordination of the muscles moving the eyes is disturbed, the affected person will have double vision. Because the eyes are not aligned properly, images on the part of each eye that senses light, the retina, will not project to equivalent areas in the brain. The brain sees two images because the same image seems to be coming from two different sources. The eyes do not agree on the source unless their movements are synchronized.

This double vision is often nauseating and always disabling. Walking, reaching, and other movements will be disturbed by the altered vision. The simplest solution to this problem is to patch one eye. With only one eye at work, there can be only one image. If movements are more impaired in one eye than the other, it is most helpful to patch the eye with the better coordination. If the alignment of the eyes is disturbed by a constant amount, the misalignment can be compensated for with special lenses called prisms. The prism bends the light to bring it into the eye at an angle that compensates for the abnormal position of the eye.

Double vision developing because of multiple sclerosis is generally not a persistent problem. It usually develops with flare-ups and subsides completely as the flare-up abates. No long-term adjustments are necessary. The patch or prisms can usually be discarded after a few days or weeks.

Moving Images

At times, some individuals with multiple sclerosis have the illusion of movement in the environment. They see objects moving that are not actually moving. This can be dangerous for someone operating a motor vehicle or other machinery that will not simply stop when the operator loses control.

Illusory movement may develop in people with the involuntary, jerking movements of the eyes called nystagmus, but that the eyes move uncontrollably does not mean that the environment will appear to move. In fact, most people with persistent nystagmus do not complain of illusory movement.

There is no simple technique for eliminating this symptom or reducing its impact on independent activity. Fortunately, this illusion of movement usually only develops during flare-ups and subsides over the course of days or weeks as the exacerbation abates.

Legal Disability

In the United States, an individual is considered legally blind when corrected vision (with glasses or contacts) in the better eye is poorer than 20/200 or when the extent of the visual field in the good eye is narrower than 20 degrees of arc. These technical measurements should be obtained by an optometrist or ophthalmologist. If an optometrist or ophthalmologist determines that an individual's vision is this limited, that person may qualify for disability payments and other services that are provided by state and local facilities for the visually impaired. In some states, public libraries will prepare recordings of written material for people who are legally disabled by virtue of a visual impairment. Establishing this legal disability may require considerable paperwork, much of which may be completed by local social service agencies. These agencies will also know what benefits are available to individuals who are designated legally blind. If state or provincial social service agencies are not helpful, the National Multiple Sclerosis Society may be able to help with application and benefit information.

Transportation

A qualified physician or physical therapist should determine what aids will assist in maximizing a person's mobility. The individual's own impression of what he or she is or is not able to do is often distorted by denial of problems or frustration in the face of relatively minor handicaps. It is just as destructive for someone to fall because their stability in walking was overestimated as it is for someone to be relegated to a wheelchair because leg strength was underestimated. An individual's independence must be maximized, but not at the risk of injury.

Automotive Aids

Most people with multiple sclerosis do not lose their ability to drive an automobile, and for many there are simple aids that can be used to reduce the fatigue of driving. Such automotive aids include attachments to the steering wheel that make it easier to hold or turn the wheel. This may be little more than some non-slip padding, or it may involve a ball mounted on the side of the wheel closest to the person's strongest arm so that wider excursions of the wheel can be performed with the good arm. Individuals with leg weakness or spasticity may require hand controls. Such controls do not necessarily interfere with the operation of the foot pedals, and so other people without leg problems can also use the car.

Clumsy individuals are not necessarily unable to drive. For many, the clumsiness is evident only when they try to perform fine, coordinated acts that are not involved in driving an automobile. An occupational or physical therapist can usually assess whether driving is practical for someone who feels slightly uncoordinated. A reassessment of strength and coordination should be performed every 6 months if the person with multiple sclerosis or the physician feels there has been deterioration that might interfere with driving.

Bicycles and Motorcycles

Anyone with balance problems should not attempt to drive a motorcycle or bicycle. Even if the affected person can operate such vehicles when they are on a smooth surface in an untrafficked region, the risk of injury from falling is too great. The major danger for the individual with balance problems is not being able to coordinate a fall. A normal young adult can fall off a bicycle without suffering substantial injury because his or her nervous system can adjust body position fast enough to reduce the trauma of impact. The person with damage to the balance system loses this orienting ability early and usually lands traumatically.

Self-Propelled Devices

A variety of battery-powered vehicles are available to assist individuals who are unable to stand and have insufficient strength in their arms to use a conventional wheelchair. Electric carts with seats that rotate for easy mounting and dismounting and steering gears that require little side-to-side arm movement for effective control are widely available (Figure 9–1). Most of these are accessible to even the most financially limited people with multiple sclerosis because they are covered by such insurance plans as Medicare or state-assisted health programs.

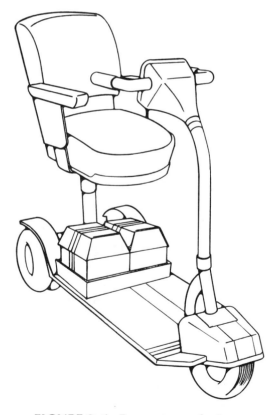

FIGURE 9–1. *Battery-powered tricart.*

Diet and Drugs

Modifications may be needed in what an individual eats if specific complications of multiple sclerosis appear. An adequate amount of calories, vitamins, and essential fatty acids always must be included in the diet to minimize disabilities. If the risk of pressure sores is high, the individual must be provided with enough calories to avoid any loss of weight. If the person is inactive and overweight, the diet must be adjusted to reduce weight and thereby reduce the added burden imposed on the impaired nervous system.

Obesity

People with severe limitation of activity will gain weight if no change is made in their diets. Walking may use up few calories, but sitting uses many fewer. The person with a flare-up of disease or with progressive leg weakness can quickly gain weight. If he or she is being treated with ACTH or steroids, this is even more likely. The added weight imposes extra burdens on the nervous system simply because it takes more nervous system control to move a heavy limb than a light one or to balance a heavy trunk rather than a slim one.

The simplest measures to avoid obesity are to increase activity as much as is practical and to restrict calories as much as is tolerable. With limited activity, food may become as much a distraction as other types of entertainment, but the long-term disadvantages of excess weight are substantial. When movement is severely limited, pressure sores develop more easily in the obese individual. If simply restricting food intake has no effect on the person's increasing girth, consultation with an experienced nutritionist is advisable. The nutritionist can estimate the number of calories being consumed daily from the type and amount of food consumed and make specific recommendations on which types of foods to eliminate and which to increase.

Exercise should not be neglected because the individual is unsteady or even unable to walk. Arm exercise with small barbells and trunk exercises against stationary objects can improve muscle tone, increase lung and heart reserves, and burn up calories. For the individual with substantial limb weakness, a physical therapist should be involved in developing the exercises so that no damage is done to surfaces or joints that are used. Swimming is especially useful for anyone who can safely participate in this type of activity.

Weight-Reducing Diets

If a weight-reducing diet is imposed, it must be designed to very gradually reduce weight. It is obviously reasonable to try to rapidly minimize the weight of an individual unable to transfer himself out of bed or into chairs, but weight loss involves dietary stress, and dietary stress is as potentially disabling for the person with multiple sclerosis as is any other stress. In the obese individual, weight itself may play a major role in the production of pressure sores, but even in that situation, the urgency to lose weight must be kept in the perspective of an equally urgent need to maintain good nutrition. The obese individual with paraplegia and contractures cannot be placed on a restricted caloric intake simply because this weight-reducing regimen will lower the individual's resistance to pressure injuries. Any weight-reducing diet adopted should be designed with the help of a nutritionist familiar with neurologic problems.

Alcohol

Changes in alcohol tolerance may develop with multiple sclerosis, and so consumption of beverages high in alcohol should be limited to whatever level produces no substantial impairment. Just because someone could drink six cans of beer before he or she developed the neurologic problem does not mean that that person will be able to tolerate even two cans of beer during a flare-up of the disease. The person with multiple sclerosis need not avoid all alcohol, but he or she should realize that alcohol tolerance must be periodically reassessed.

It is best if the affected individual does not drink alcoholic beverages at all. Alcohol places extra burdens on the nervous system, and so drinking must be kept to a minimum. The balance system in the cerebellum is especially vulnerable to the effects of alcohol. Even a nonintoxicating amount of alcohol will interfere with coordination if the cerebellum is impaired by demyelination. Chronic alcohol excess damages the nerve cells in the cerebellum and, to a lesser extent, cells in other parts of the brain. This damage, even if it is minor, will have a major impact on the person with underlying cerebellar disease. Slurred speech, difficulty with walking, and problems with handwriting will appear after consumption of a relatively small amount of alcohol. Coordination impairments will be out of proportion to intellectual impairment, and so the individual with multiple sclerosis may find that it is unsafe to drive after drinking a very small amount of alcohol even though his or her thinking is still clear.

Illicit Drugs

All drugs that an individual takes must be evaluated in terms of the effects they have on the nervous system, but this is especially true of illicit drugs. There is no good documentation that any of the widely used recreational drugs, such as marijuana and cocaine, cause irreversible problems for the person with multiple sclerosis, but risks are inherent in using any illicit drug. By the very nature of the substance, the individual cannot know what he is actually taking. Marijuana can be tainted with herbicides or insecticides that are devastating for the person with nervous system impairment. Cocaine is routinely "cut" or adulterated with a wide array of agents that can stress even the intact nervous system and can cause very serious reactions in the damaged nervous system. Blood pressure regulation and heart activity, for instance, can be dangerously impaired by some of the stimulants and anesthetic agents commonly used to "cut" cocaine.

Morphine, heroin, and meperidine (Demerol) addiction are no less a problem for the individual with multiple sclerosis than they are for persons without demyelinating disease. Indeed, addiction to narcotics is often more a complication of medical treatment for chronically impaired individuals than for individuals with nonchronic, nonpainful disorders. The person with painful contractures may appropriately be treated with liberal doses of these narcotics, but the physician and the patient must take care that the drug does not become as much a problem as the spasms for which it was given.

Clothing

Barriers to independent lifestyles are built into both the clothing and housing available to most people with moderate disabilities. One of the major lifestyle adjustments for the person with multiple sclerosis is recognizing these barriers and developing strategies or equipment to overcome them. Most of the changes appropriate for the individual who is only slightly impaired involve little or no expense and may amount to nothing more than modifications in habits. People with severe disabilities, on the other hand, may need to make substantial changes in their homes and habits.

Something as simple as a button may be impractical for the person with severe coordination difficulties. Button loops, devices that allow the button to be caught and pulled through the buttonhole with one hand, simplify the task for individuals with weakness or poor coordination. Wherever possible, buttons should be eliminated if they present barriers to easy dressing. If buttons are used, they should be large (that is, greater than 5/8 inch in diameter) and textured in some way to simplify handling.

Materials such as Velcro can be substituted for other types of fastening devices on clothing. Even shoes are available with Velcro fasteners or elastic loops to hold them securely to the foot. Problems with shoes, boots, or other types of footwear that are not easily put on are common for individuals with coordination problems. With lower leg spasticity or weakness, the individual will profit from using such aids as shoe horns with long handles. Those who drag a foot when they try to walk should use shoes with smooth soles to minimize friction on rugs and other surfaces that impede the movement of textured soles.

Elastic waistbands and multiple concealed zippers may simplify dressing. With elastic materials, the pressure exerted on the skin should be minimal. Tightly fitting garments may produce discomfort for the person who cannot shift his or her weight easily and may cause pressure sores in people with impaired sensation.

Regardless of what type of clothing the individual chooses to wear, it should not interfere with free movement. Tightly fitting clothes hinder the person with spasticity or weakness. Loosely fitting garments are generally much more practical than tailored or restrictive clothing. For women, wrap-around clothing may be both practical and fashionable. Pockets are usually not useful for the person with hand weakness or clumsiness. An easily opening bag or pouch provides greater access to belongings than a pocket and reduces the risk of losing items that are pulled out of a pocket unintentionally.

Clothing choices should also take into consideration requirements imposed by bowel and bladder habits. The man with poor coordination should not have to struggle with zippers and buttons every time he has to urinate. Women with poor bladder control and impaired grip should opt for dresses and skirts, rather than pants or shorts, when they are traveling, so that undressing to urinate becomes simpler. Restricting girdles are likely to be uncomfortable and impractical for the person with incontinence, because pressure on the abdomen will worsen the control problem and the extra clothing will interfere with efforts to urinate or defecate.

Housing

Modifications in housing and work places, like those for clothing, must take into account the affected individual's abilities and disabilities. Steps bar people in wheelchairs from access to many facilities, but the growing awareness of this barrier in public places has led to increased installation of ramps. Of course, adjustments in housing may be required even if the individual is not in a wheelchair. That someone *can* climb stairs does not mean that he or she *should* climb stairs. A living area limited to a single level may save enough energy for the affected person to accomplish much more in terms of independent activities. A single-level dwelling is especially valuable for the person who is largely dependent on a wheelchair. Various types of lifting devices are available for people dependent on wheelchairs, but these are fairly expensive and require skilled installation.

Many of the common barriers built into housing can be eliminated with little expense and effort. The thresholds between rooms or at the entrance of living areas can be flattened to simplify movement through doorways. If doors do not open widely enough, they can be remounted with 180-degree hinges, which will allow the door to swing completely clear of the doorway. Eliminating the width of the door from the doorway with this type of hinge provides only an extra inch or two of space, but this may allow wheelchair access that would not otherwise be possible.

Ramps can be installed to replace single steps. The ramps should be wide enough to allow someone with a four-legged walker or wheelchair to maneuver with safety, and that generally means a ramp at least 3, but preferably 4, feet wide. Every 1 inch of step height requires about 1 foot of ramp length, and so an 8-inch step would be most easily overcome if the ramp were 7 to 8 feet in length. If something must be done at the top of the ramp, such as unlocking a door, modifications of the area should take into account the need to maneuver on a flat surface.

Someone with a walker or in a wheelchair cannot safely maneuver on an inclined surface, and so the ramp cannot end at the point where the individual needs to have an unencumbered grip. At a doorway with a locked door or at a point where a change in direction is required, an uninclined platform that is at least 3 feet by 3 feet should be installed for the person with a walker, and one at least 3 feet by 4 feet for the person in a wheelchair.

Grab bars should be installed on the walls wherever extra stability is needed. This is especially likely to be required in bathrooms and kitchens. Only grab bars specifically designed to support the full weight of the impaired individual should be used. If the individual has a poor grip, high-friction materials can be applied to the bars to reduce the risk of falls. Places where bars should always be installed, even if the affected person has only moderate weakness or instability, are in showers and baths, alongside toilets, and at sinks. An occupational therapist or other individual skilled in the arrangement of home health aids should be involved in the selection and installation of the necessary materials.

Kitchen Aids

Ideally, the kitchen should be designed to take into account the limitations of the person using it. This means adjusting counter heights, installing appliances with special safety features, using rotating and adjustable shelves, and eliminating unreachable space. For most people with multiple sclerosis, it is not financially practical to design and build a kitchen with all the space and safety measures needed. Consequently, efforts should be made to reduce the dangers in the kitchen as much as possible, even if convenience cannot be increased.

Automatic appliances, such as dishwashers, can openers, and trash compactors are enormous aids for people with limited mobility and coordination. If the individual wishes to cook, counter-top burners ideally should be arranged in a single row so that there is no need to reach over a hot burner. Cooking utensils should have easily grasped handles and extra insulation to protect the poorly coordinated person against burns. Storage space should be planned at a height and depth that cause no problems with access. Shelves that pull out or rotate should be used wherever possible to avoid the need to reach around obstacles.

Narrow double doors on a refrigerator are simple to manage and require less clearance than a single wide door. This is of special importance to the person who is confined to a wheelchair and must manage the wheelchair while opening the door. Refrigerators with freezing compartments that are low or upright are more practical than those with high compartments if the person has difficulty standing or reaching. The individual with weakness, sensory impairment, or clumsiness must be guarded against frostbite. Freezing injuries can occur in seconds. Protective mittens should be within easy reach of the freezer and should be worn routinely even if the affected person is fairly confident of his or her strength and coordination.

Bedroom Aids

Adjustments to accommodate handicaps are usually more feasible in the bedroom than in the kitchen. The height of the bed can usually be lowered or raised by cutting the legs or mounting the bed on blocks. The most accessible height is determined by trial and error. If the person with multiple sclerosis has difficulty changing position in bed, a number of strategies may be adopted to increase comfort and reduce the risk of pressure sores. A lamb's-wool covering under skin surfaces that are subject to the most pressure is the simplest precaution against injury, but many people need more substantial reductions in local pressure. A water mattress is often helpful, but the major limitation of this type of surface is that it is quite difficult to change position on a water mattress. Textured surface material, such as foam "egg crating," may provide a sufficient compromise.

Bathroom Aids

Adjustments are required in bathing and toileting if the individual has sensory, movement, or coordination problems. The more impaired the individual, the greater the need for environmental adjustments. People with minor problems should not, however, dismiss their limitations. Ignoring deficiencies invites accidents. The person with impaired temperature sense alone is more likely to end up with burns because of excessively hot water in the shower or bath than is the person with numerous other problems. The more impaired individual is more obliged to be cautious and

so is more likely to be conscientious in guarding against accidental injury.

Avoiding Burns

In any bathroom or shower facility, the person with multiple
sclerosis must be aware of the danger of burns from hot water or
unshielded pipes carrying hot water. A variety of inexpensive,
unbreakable thermometers can be used by individuals with good
vision to monitor water temperature. For those with poor vision,
more expensive digital devices that display the temperature in
large numbers are available. These larger devices are less conven-
ient to carry about, although they are portable and are usually no
larger than a carton of cigarettes. Medical supply houses routinely
carry several different types of thermometers. If the individual
uses the same bath facility on a regular basis, the thermometer
should be mounted in a position that provides good visibility and
adequate immersion in the water of the bath, sink, or shower.
Where possible, reducing the water heater setting is another
safety measure.

Individuals with impaired walking must identify all exposed
hot water pipes and scrupulously avoid or effectively insulate
them. People in wheelchairs must be especially careful of pipes
below sinks; these pipes do not feel hot until they start carrying
hot water. Any modifications in the sink that allow a wheelchair to
slip under it must be accompanied by adequate insulation of the
hot-water pipes.

Modifications in the bathroom accessories should take into
account all limitations of the person with multiple sclerosis. If he
or she is wheelchair bound, toiletries should be within easy reach
on shelves placed in unobstructed areas. A low mirror or mirrors
on flexible bases will simplify shaving and make-up application for
one with limited mobility.

Installing Grab Bars and Rails

Most bathrooms are not designed for people with impaired walking or balance, so most must be modified to make them safe if

they are being used by people with multiple sclerosis. As already mentioned, grab bars are essential elements in the bathroom near the toilet, sink, bath, and shower. These bars must be firmly anchored on wall supports and not simply attached to the plaster or tile by plastic or lead anchors. All unstable or breakable items protruding from the walls should be removed. This means that glass or plastic towel racks and glass shelving must be removed.

Grab bars are ideally made of tubular metal or high-strength plastic, but much less expensive and equally effective are properly installed wooden rails. These rails can be fastened to the wall studs by metal brackets and painted to match the decor of the bathroom. Because they cost much less than metal or plastic bars, they may be used along the entire length of the bathroom walls at little additional expense. More specialized grab bars that attach directly to the bathtub are available.

Modifying Doorways

In addition to grab bars, modifications should include simplified access to the bathing facilities. The first barrier for the person with difficulty in walking is the doorway. Many houses and apartments have narrower doors on the bathrooms than on the other rooms. For someone using a walker, the doorway should be at least 32 inches wide; for someone in a wheelchair, it should be 35 inches wide. If the bathroom is approached by a hallway, that space should be at least 42 inches wide to allow easy maneuvering of a wheelchair at the entrance to the bathroom.

If the doorway cannot be altered, there may be advantages in changing or remounting the door. For people who do not need privacy, the door may simply be removed. Light, swinging doors can provide privacy and yet not present substantial obstacles to entry. Some people may want the privacy provided by a more substantial door that can be fastened shut, in which case the direction in which the door swings may be revised. Most bathroom doors open into the bathroom, whereas most impaired individuals find it more practical to deal with doors that open out of the bathroom. The more confined space of the bathroom makes the door an additional obstacle if it must be pulled into the room when exiting.

These types of modifications are not expensive, but they may be impractical for the person who rents housing. The landlord is likely to object to structural changes in the property. In that case, the individual who is wheelchair bound will find it helpful to use a commode chair with wheels that can be left just inside the entrance to the bathroom. At the entrance, he or she transfers to the commode and uses that for moving about the bathroom. This has the disadvantage of being less easily moved than a wheelchair, but with wooden rails about the perimeter of the bathroom most people with enough arm strength to transfer themselves onto the commode chair will be able to move themselves about the bathroom.

Choosing Sinks

The appropriate type of sink depends on whether or not the affected individual must be seated. Even people who are not dependent on walkers or wheelchairs may find it wise to sit when washing, shaving, or applying make-up. A little instability can produce a serious fall if the person closes his or her eyes while washing and there is no wall to lean against. The sink should have no vanity underneath it to interfere with sitting or wheeling up to the sink on a commode or wheelchair. A reasonable height for the sink is 30 inches. As already mentioned, pipes beneath the sink must be well-insulated to avoid burns on the legs.

Sink fixtures should be tailored to the affected person's level of coordination and strength. Faucets are usually easiest to open and close if they have large lever-type handles. The nozzle may have swivel attachments to help direct the water. Any racks placed near the sink should be unbreakable, free of sharp edges, and mounted at a level that provides easy access. A low cabinet may be more feasible than a set of shelves. A medicine cabinet over the sink is of no use to someone who cannot stand without support. The narrow shelves of typical medicine cabinets are also impractical for someone with impaired coordination or tremors.

Any medication kept in the bathroom should be clearly marked, and efforts should be made to safeguard it from children. Limiting children's access to these drugs while providing easy access for the disabled person may require some ingenuity, but it is important, even if children visit the living quarters only occasionally. An inexpensive, but child-resistant, barrier is a latch that yields when the door it is securing is pushed upon, rather than pulled upon. Discovering how this type of door opens may take enough time to allow detection of the child's action. A buzzer or other type of alarm can be installed where medications are stored if there are young children living in the house or apartment with the person taking medication.

Choosing Showers and Tubs

Bathtubs are usually not practical for people with limited coordination or poor strength. Ideally, the tub should be replaced with a large shower stall (Figure 9–2). If that is not financially practical, then safety measures must be taken to avoid injuries in the tub. Securely anchored, horizontal grab bars or rails should be on the walls surrounding the tub. Nonskid materials should be outside and inside the tub, so that the individual will be less likely to slip or fall while climbing into or out of the tub. A hand-held showering device or water massage is best for the person with enough hand and arm coordination to use it properly (Figure 9–3). A single-lever faucet is simpler to operate than two conventional faucets and is usually no more expensive than conventional faucets. This type of fixture will require special installation by a plumber.

People who are dependent on wheelchairs can simplify their transfer to the bathtub by getting a bench that extends over the edge of the bathtub, as shown in Figure 9–3. After getting onto the bench from the wheelchair, the person swings both legs over to be properly positioned.

Regardless of how the bath is revised, a shower stall is always preferable. It should have a shower curtain, rather than a shower door. If there is a step up to the shower, this should be modified

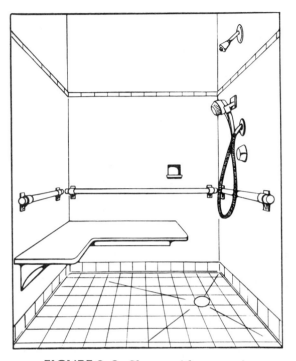

FIGURE 9–2. *Shower with accessories.*

with a ramp. Slip-resistant materials installed in the shower or bath help prevent falls, but more practical measures for people with problems in walking include shower chairs and bath chairs. Showering can be greatly simplified if the individual can move the shower head, rather than moving himself or herself, while washing. Hose-mounted shower heads are inexpensive and can be easily interchanged with conventional fixed shower heads with no plumbing expertise whatsoever.

If hand coordination or grip strength is a problem, devices for easing the person's hold on soap and scrubbing materials are available. Scrubbing gloves and scrubbing brushes with extension poles can help the individual reach all parts of the body readily. Suction devices to hold soap and other slippery shower and bath materials can be purchased in medical supply houses.

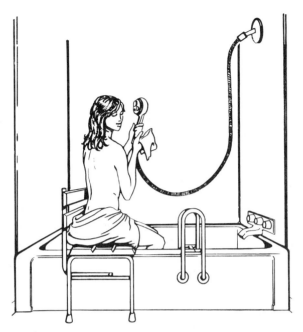

FIGURE 9–3. *Bath modifications for showering.*

Toileting

The most practical toilet for an individual dependent on a wheelchair is one that is mounted on the wall, rather than the floor, at a height that simplifies transfer off the wheelchair. Standard floor-mounted toilets are too low for easy transfer, but raised seats are available for standard toilets, so that extensive plumbing changes are not necessary in most living quarters. For the very unsteady person, raised seats with armrests are available. Whether the affected individual is unable to walk or simply unsteady when changing positions, grab bars should be installed beside the toilet to ease transfer on and off the toilet seat.

Some individuals with impaired hand coordination cannot use toilet paper. If it is financially practical, these people are best served by installing a bidet, which is a device to wash the anal region. If this is not practical, alternatives must be developed to keep the individual clean after urination or bowel movements.

Shaving

Anyone with impaired coordination, tremor, or a weak grip should use an electric razor if he or she chooses to shave. A straight razor is a potentially lethal tool, and a safety razor provides little additional protection. The most easily manipulated shaving device is a cordless electric razor. These are available commercially and are relatively inexpensive.

Dental Care

The fine coordination required for adequate dental care is often beyond the capability of even mildly uncoordinated people. Fortunately, there are effective alternatives to toothbrushes and dental floss. A water pick, that is, a device that drives a fine, pulsed stream of water between the teeth at high pressure, requires some patience, but very little coordination or strength. These are commercially available and require no special plumbing.

CHAPTER 10

Rehabilitation

Rehabilitation is the technique used to recover lost strength, skills, or coordination. With any illness that interferes with neurologic function, rehabilitation may be effective. This is especially true with multiple sclerosis because the neurologic disease is not necessarily progressive. Between flare-ups, much of the weakness, speech difficulty, or incoordination that developed with the flare-up can be compensated for with physical or occupational therapy. The principal goal of rehabilitation for the person with multiple sclerosis is to maximize his or her abilities. Mobility, speech, and independence may all be improved with proper management.

Some problems, such as vision loss or sensory changes, are not affected by attempts at retraining. Bladder control may fail to improve despite efforts to increase voluntary control over bladder emptying, but incontinence may be minimized with changes in the timing of fluid intake and of visits to the toilet. The neurologic disturbances most readily helped by treatment are those involving weakness in the arms and legs.

When Does Multiple Sclerosis Disappear?

Rehabilitation will not affect when multiple sclerosis stops being a problem. Therapy will help to reduce the burdens imposed by the disease, but the disease itself will abate whether the person with multiple sclerosis receives therapy or not. Although the damage done to the nervous system may not completely reverse even after the disease has been silent for decades, the individual can expect new symptoms of the disease to stop appearing in time. Multiple sclerosis is primarily a disease of young adults, and this is one of the justifications for aggressive physical and occupational therapy when the disease no longer appears to be active.

The violent exacerbations of disease that occur in an affected person's late teens and early twenties are less likely to occur in his or her thirties. If little damage has occurred from the flare-ups before a person reaches 30 years of age, he or she may enter middle age virtually unimpaired by the disease. If deficits, whether they are minor or major, have persisted after exacerbations in early adult life, the disease is more likely to enter a chronic, progressive phase as the person ages. The tendency to have flare-ups decreases with age, but the tendency to have remissions also decreases. This means that a severe episode of multiple sclerosis is less likely when one is 30 years old than when one is 20 years old, but complete relief from symptoms of the disease is also less likely.

People who develop multiple sclerosis in their thirties and forties are much less likely to exhibit the typical pattern of relapses and remissions. Statistically, the outlook for these individuals is worse than for the younger person with multiple sclerosis. The disease progresses and produces handicaps that do not go away. Physical therapy may compensate for some of the handicaps that develop, but rehabilitation efforts with this type of disease are most useful if they focus on occupational therapy to retrain the individual to achieve greater independent functioning.

With the complications that may develop with severe multiple sclerosis, some decrease in life expectancy is unavoidable, but it is relatively slight. Of men diagnosed as having multiple sclerosis, 76 percent are alive 20 years after the onset of the disease, and 70 percent are alive 25 years after the onset. If both men and women are considered together, the overall 25-year survival after multiple sclerosis becomes symptomatic is 74 percent. This is less than the expected survival rate of 86 percent, but it is not dramatically less.

This survival is not simply that of a severely impaired individual. Although the ability to walk is often impaired in people with this illness, at least 65 percent of those with multiple sclerosis who survive 25 years with the disease are still able to walk, regardless of what treatment they receive. The outlook for the individual with multiple sclerosis is statistically good, if good is defined in terms of leading a relatively independent life with little disturbance from neurologic disease.

Physical Therapy

During an exacerbation, changes in muscle strength and coordination develop that may be as much from the inactivity imposed by the flare-up as from the neurologic damage inflicted. Not being able to move a limb results in muscle loss and lessened coordination of muscle action. Even after the unused muscle recovers the nervous system back-up necessary for normal function, it still fails to do all that it can because it is simply out of shape and out of practice. The individual usually does not realize what the true capacity of the limb is and often assumes that the abilities that were impaired during the flare-up will remain impaired. Retraining the limb with the assistance of a skilled physical therapist may restore much or all of its original strength and coordination.

Unfortunately, many individuals with a high potential for recovery of strength and coordination cannot tolerate the therapy required to regain those abilities. The susceptibility to fatigue that develops as a sign of multiple sclerosis interferes with their therapy. Even when the nervous system has recovered adequately to allow normal muscle function, the affected person may still fatigue easily. Increasing the level of activity when fatigue is a major problem is unwise because it unduly increases the individual's stress.

Timing of Therapy

During a flare-up of multiple sclerosis, the affected person ultimately fares better if he or she is simply allowed to rest for a few days. Increasing the use of an arm or leg as the strength or

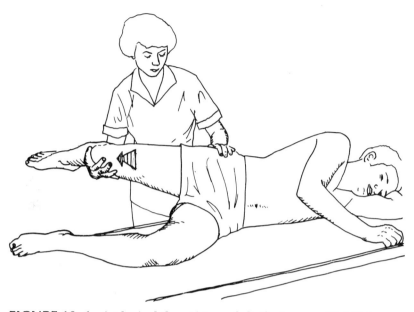

FIGURE 10–1. *A physical therapist can help the person with MS to move paralyzed limbs, avoiding contractures and degeneration of joints. Here, the hip is extended toward the back. (From Kisner, C and Colby, LA: Therapeutic Exercise: Foundations and Techniques, ed 2. FA Davis, Philadelphia, 1990, p 35, with permission.)*

coordination in that limb deteriorates does not shorten the time required for recovery of function in that limb. Pushing an individual to walk at the time when he or she is developing progressive leg weakness is not useful. When the neurologic deterioration has stabilized and no new signs are appearing, therapy should be started. At first, little more need be done than encouraging movement in the affected limbs. If the limb is paralyzed, the individual will still benefit from manipulation of the limb by a physical therapist. The joints will be kept from degenerating, and the contractures developing because of spasticity in the affected limb will be limited (Figure 10–1).

The pace of the therapy will be determined by what the affected person can safely tolerate and what the therapist considers reasonable goals. If the individual lacks self-confidence, the physical therapist will be a better judge of how aggressive the therapy should be. If the affected person is unrealistic about his limitations, the therapist can help limit the goals that the individual should expect to achieve.

Design of the Therapy Program

The most important goals in physical therapy are increasing strength and endurance. Strength in an individual muscle may respond to repeated efforts to lift maximum loads, but endurance requires the increasingly frequent repetition of an activity in which the muscle group exercised faces little or no weight load or resistance.

When any part of the body is exercised, other parts of the body may be strained. Lifting weights with the arms will place demands on the shoulders and the spine, and what these indirectly involved body parts can stand must be considered in the design of any exercise program. Back problems will develop if the spine is strained during arm or leg exercises. Back problems may even develop if posture or the manner of walking is faulty. Standing and walking make demands on the spine if coordination of the muscles supporting the spine is inadequate. This means that in any therapy program designed to help the person with multiple sclerosis to walk, constant attention must be paid to developing the strength and alignment of the muscles in the back as well as in the legs, thighs, and hips.

All exercise regimens should be performed in a relatively cool environment because of the effect of heat on the impaired nervous system. As already discussed, heat worsens the severity of apparent deficits and may produce additional problems with strength and coordination. These are transient problems that remit when the individual cools off.

Water Therapy

Physical therapy performed in water is especially useful for people with extreme limitations of mobility. The water produces resistance to movement without the destructive effects on impaired joints that typically occur with weight-bearing exercises. Pools designed for physical therapy have ramps or other access devices that allow people in wheelchairs to enter them safely. In the water, a therapist can help the individual increase limb flexibility, range of motion, and physical independence. With the increased activity, muscle tone will often improve.

Continuing Therapy

Because the physical impairments of individuals with MS are likely to develop asymmetrically, abnormal postures are a constant problem. This means that activities and exercises directed at counteracting the altered posture must be used by the affected person on a regular basis for a prolonged period. Stretching exercises that push joints close to their full range of motion should be included in any exercise regimen adopted. This type of exercise must be continued daily, even when the person no longer has access to supervision.

For the severely impaired, the use of mechanical aids becomes an important part of any therapy program. Polyethylene short leg braces (as shown in Figure 7–2) may compensate for a footdrop, but the individual needs to be trained to walk with the brace. With more severe problems, he or she may need a four-legged walker.

Much of the exercise and discipline required to maintain optimal limb strength and coordination must be done by the individual without supervision. A therapist can provide supervision for only a few hours a day at most, and most people do not need the expensive and usually uncomfortable environment of a hospital or rehabilitation facility to continue their recovery. Unfortunately, many become inactive when they are unsupervised. Depression limits their initiative, and early fatigue blunts their enthusiasm. Continued participation in a rehabilitation program or enrollment in a rehabilitation facility will produce better long-term results than depending on the individual's undirected efforts at home. Even after the person goes home, physical therapy performed by a professional is essential as long as significant problems with strength and spasticity persist.

Occupational Therapy

With occupational therapy, the person with severe limitations can learn how to simplify activities encountered in routine daily life. The occupational therapist also helps with adjustments in recreation, and can make recommendations on how to modify the home environment to make it easier for the person with multiple sclerosis to function. Specific recommendations for changes in the home are discussed in Chapter 9.

Psychological Support

The unpredictability of multiple sclerosis produces special stresses for affected individuals. Those affected are usually at a stage in their lives when they are making long-term plans. They must decide whether or not to have children, what kind of work to pursue, and what kinds of relationships to form. The uncertainty surrounding what the long-term effects of the multiple sclerosis will be undermines much of this planning. The most important service the person's family and friends can provide is intelligent assistance. The person with multiple sclerosis should not become the focus for all the family's efforts, nor should he or she be the ultimate recipient of all the family's resources.

Overwhelming the affected individual with attention and assistance is as destructive as abandonment. A lifestyle as close to normal as possible should be sought. The affected individual should be allowed and encouraged to contribute to the family in whatever ways are practical. If the person has few or no apparent problems, the contribution should be unaffected by the threat of disease. That problems may develop is not a reasonable basis for special treatment.

Some people with multiple sclerosis exploit the problems caused by the disease or, alternatively, deny them. Family and friends must feel free to criticize the person when he or she becomes unrealistic about the actual problems caused by the multiple sclerosis, and the affected person must be prepared to adjust his or her behavior in response to that criticism. For most people, this type of exchange is most easily conducted in a group setting with similarly affected families involved as sympathetic advisers. Various local and national organizations, such as the National Multiple Sclerosis Society, conduct groups for affected people and for their families. These serve as a valuable forum in which family problems can be explored and resolved.

CHAPTER 11

Research Efforts

R esearch continues into the cause of multiple sclerosis and how the disease might be prevented, controlled, or reversed. Much of this research effort still focuses primarily on the immune system and its relationship to disease. That the investigation of the immune system has yet to reveal the basis for multiple sclerosis or a cure has prompted some researchers to look elsewhere. Rather than assuming that multiple sclerosis is an autoimmune disease in which myelin is destroyed, some research has pursued the possibility that it is a disease of the oligodendrocytes, the myelin-producing cells in the central nervous system. That a virus is involved in the attack on the myelin, on the oligodendrocyte, or on some other element of the nervous system is still considered a possibility and is still the basis for some of the ongoing research in institutions studying multiple sclerosis.

Much of the more widely publicized research has had little impact on the diagnosis or treatment of multiple sclerosis. Such highly publicized attempts as vitamin therapy and hyperbaric oxygen therapy received an enormous amount of misleading attention before their ineffectiveness could be demonstrated. The

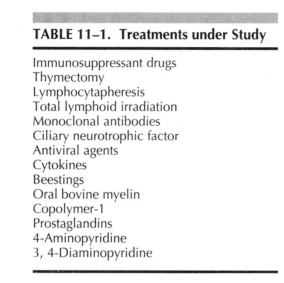

TABLE 11–1. Treatments under Study

Immunosuppressant drugs
Thymectomy
Lymphocytapheresis
Total lymphoid irradiation
Monoclonal antibodies
Ciliary neurotrophic factor
Antiviral agents
Cytokines
Beestings
Oral bovine myelin
Copolymer-1
Prostaglandins
4-Aminopyridine
3, 4-Diaminopyridine

receptiveness of people suffering from a chronic, incurable illness to any suggestion of effectiveness has been played on both inadvertently and intentionally since multiple sclerosis was first recognized as a disease. Avenues of research that authentically hold promise of advances include investigations into malfunctions of the immune system and unusual infections of the nervous system (Table 11–1). These may prove to be two aspects of the same problem.

The Immune System

The immune system protects the body against infections and rejects material that does not belong in the body. If multiple sclerosis develops because of a problem with this system, it could be from a disturbance in any one of several parts of this complex defense mechanism. Investigations over the past few decades have revealed that such mainstays of the immune reaction as the white blood cells may have altered function in multiple sclerosis. These investigations have led to promising work with immunosuppressants and antibodies.

T-Lymphocyte Function

The body's defenses are dependent on white blood cell activity, among other things. One type of white blood cell that appears to be central in the evolution of multiple sclerosis is the T lymphocyte (or T cell), a cell instrumental in the immune system reactions that lead to the breakdown of myelin. In multiple sclerosis plaques, there are scavenger cells, called macrophages, and T lymphocytes. The lymphocytes are mostly identical and are of a type that influences the manufacture of antibodies. These T cells enter the nervous system quickly at the time of an acute flare-up. They cross into the central nervous system from the bloodstream and collect in the areas of demyelination. Which occurs first, the accumulation of T cells in limited areas of the brain or the demyelination, is still not known.

Once these lymphocytes and macrophages are in regions of active disease, they interact with the myelin around nerve fibers. Some investigators are currently working with antibodies to elements of the T lymphocytes that interfere with their action against myelin. This interference has been effective in stopping demyelination in animal experiments, but it has not yet been proven useful in treating people with multiple sclerosis.

Iron is essential for the production of lymphocytes by the body. Interfering with the way the body uses iron should alter lymphocyte production and thereby limit the damage that lymphocytes inflict on the myelin sheath. Desferrioxamine, an agent that depletes iron from the body, has affected the course of demyelination in experiments with animals. This approach has obvious limitations since lymphocytes are an essential part of the body's defense system, and a severe depletion of lymphocytes, caused by reduced iron, will leave the person susceptible to infection.

The real disorder in multiple sclerosis may be inappropriate lymphocyte activity, rather than excessive activity. The T lymphocytes may be acting destructively because they are diseased. In some viral illnesses, T lymphocytes are attacked, with the result that they are destroyed or their function is disturbed. If a virus that causes lymphocytes to start the chain of events leading to demyelination can be identified, a vaccine against this virus could be developed.

Monoclonal Antibodies

As mentioned before, proteins produced by the body as part of the attack on foreign substances are called *antibodies*. Antibodies to one or a few closely related targets are called *monoclonal antibodies*. In experiments using animals, monoclonal antibodies directed against lymphocytes have been used to stop demyelination, and the results have been promising. Recent studies have been done with humans using antibodies produced by mice, which were directed against specific populations of the antibody-promoting T cells. Patients responded to these monoclonal antibodies by showing less antibody production. Whether or not this will affect the outcome of progressive multiple sclerosis remains to be seen.

New Agents That Block Immune Responses

Because there is considerable evidence that multiple sclerosis is caused by a disturbance, if not indeed a defect, in the immune system, studies continue with conventional and newly developed agents that block or inhibit immune responses (immunosuppressant agents). Cyclophosphamide (Cytoxan) has been widely used in people with multiple sclerosis and some researchers are encouraged by the results. New studies will be attempted using periodically repeated doses of cyclophosphamide every 2 months to see if transient slowing of disease progression in the chronic progressive form of multiple sclerosis can be continued with repeated exposure to the medication. Low-dose azathioprine (Imuran) and methotrexate, immunosuppressant agents that can be taken by mouth, also look promising in some studies of people with chronic progressive multiple sclerosis.

Total irradiation (exposure to intense x-rays) of the body's lymphoid tissue is probably impractical because it exposes an individual to risk of infection, but some modification of this approach may prove useful. Studies using total lymphoid irradiation have been conducted over the course of several years, and the researchers believe the technique has considerable promise.

Cytokines

The immune system is regulated at least in part by substances called **cytokines.** Interferons are one type of cytokine; **interleukins** are another. Many of these regulatory substances are made by cells of the immune system, such as the T cells and macrophages. The cytokines of individuals with multiple sclerosis show a variety of changes, but many, if not all, of the changes are effects, rather than causes, of demyelinating disease. That beta interferon has a beneficial effect in some patients with multiple sclerosis and gamma interferon has a negative effect suggests that altering various cytokines may affect the course of the disease.

There is also evidence that cytokines may have a much more direct effect on central nervous system tissues. In studies of fish, damage to the optic nerve initiated a chain of events that led to destruction of oligodendrocytes, the cells that make myelin. The injury to the nerve fibers caused an enzyme to bond two inter-leukin (IL-2) molecules together. This new molecule injured the oligodendrocytes in the optic nerve. Destruction of the oligoden-drocytes in the damaged area was followed by clearing away of the myelin produced by these cells. The severed nerve fibers were able to regrow and repair only after this demyelination had occured. Demyelination appears to be part of the mechanism by which the optic nerve is repaired in these fish.

Although this process in fish may have nothing to do with multiple sclerosis, there is an alternative view that this type of attack by cytokines plays a role in human demyelinating disease. According to this view, an agent such as a virus periodically breaks through the immune defense system of the central nervous system and triggers the formation (in small areas) of cytokines that injure other cells, similar to the paired IL-2 molecules in the fish. Possibly, the virus causes nerve damage, simulates it, or directly triggers the enzymes that lead to the production of the damaging cytokines. These cytokines attack the oligodendrocytes, leading to demyelination by depriving the myelin sheath of the cells responsible for its maintenance and production. In this view, much of the immune reaction observed in multiple sclerosis is merely an effect, rather than a cause, of the disease. The immune system would be called on merely to clean up the damaged myelin of the injured or dying oligondendrocyte to allow new cells to move in and produce healthy myelin.

If this theory is correct, agents that could stop the formation of the damaging cytokines should improve the outlook for individuals with multiple sclerosis. Some researchers believe that this type of activity is precisely what leads to the effects observed when some individuals with multiple sclerosis are given beta interferon, but whether this theory relates in any way to the observed activity of beta interferon or whether it will lead to the development of drugs effective in the treatment of MS is nothing more than speculation.

That cytokines interact with immune cells in very specific ways has led to research into their use as immune-cell disablers or killers. Poisons bound to the cytokines may be absorbed by their target cells along with the cytokine. Alternatively, strategies may be developed to interfere with cytokine effects on target cells. Corticosteroids may exert much of their influence on the immune system by interfering with the production of certain cytokines, such as interleukin-1.

Cytokines can only attach to cells at locations on the cell surface equipped with special molecules that serve as docking sites. These highly specialized surface molecules are referred to as *binding sites*. Antibodies to the cytokine binding sites may prevent the cytokines from exerting any action on their targets. Such antibodies offer another treatment option if specific cytokines prove to be important in the nervous system damage seen with multiple sclerosis.

Beesting Therapy

Although bee venom is an unlikely medicine, some individuals claim that they have seen improvement in their disease after multiple beestings. The risks of this approach are substantial, and objective testing of this approach has not yet proved the claims. Bee venom will produce potentially fatal reactions in a small percentage of the population, but this is precisely because it has an impact on the immune system. Current speculation by those who endorse this approach is that the bee venom brings forth an immune response that affects the course of multiple sclerosis. Decades ago similar claims were made for an element isolated from bacterial cell walls, called *endotoxin,* which as the name suggests was highly poisonous (toxic) to humans. Whether the observations made about bee venom will be yet another dead end or will provide fresh insights into treatment options remains to be seen.

Bovine Myelin

Another highly experimental therapy is the use of **bovine myelin,** the insulating material of the cow's central nervous system. People with MS have been fed this material, and its supporters claim to have seen some benefits. The studies conducted in humans have been very limited, and the analyses have been hard pressed to demonstrate an effect in most people with multiple sclerosis. Nonetheless, the prospect of a therapy that can be taken orally is so appealing that this approach is receiving much attention.

The use of bovine myelin is based on several assumptions. One is that myelin from a cow is sufficiently similar to myelin in a human to cause the immune system to mount a reaction like the one that would occur with consumption of human myelin. Another is that absorption of digested fragments of the myelin desensitizes the immune system and thereby blunts autoimmune reactions leading to demyelination. This theory, of course, assumes that the underlying cause of multiple sclerosis is an autoimmune attack on myelin.

Ciliary Neurotrophic Factor

Because the myelin-producing cell, the oligodendrocyte, rather than the myelin sheath itself, may be the target for the agent causing multiple sclerosis, increasing attention has been directed toward identifying agents that promote survival of the oligodendrocyte. Ciliary neurotrophic factor (CNTF) promotes the survival of these cells in the laboratory, but it remains to be seen whether or not this material is useful in individuals with multiple sclerosis. CNTF occurs normally in the healthy nervous system. How CNTF protects oligodendrocytes is still open to speculation, but it is known that it helps them to resist the toxic activities of a cytokine, called *tumor necrosis factor,* which is found in increased concentration in areas of demyelination.

Antiviral Agents

Efforts to identify a virus that can be confidently linked to multiple sclerosis have been disappointing. Studies of types 1 and 2 herpes simplex, herpes zoster, measles, and Epstein-Barr viruses have all failed to relate multiple sclerosis to these common causes of viral illnesses convincingly. However, studies of viruses have not been entirely fruitless.

Several different viruses have been identified that have structures chemically similar to one of the major proteins that make up myelin. This raises the possibility that the body may be reacting to constituents of myelin. There are mechanisms built into the immune system to prevent it from committing attacks on "self," but reactions initiated by infectious agents may trigger self-destructive actions. Because of this, increasing attention is being given to specific agents such as acyclovir, a drug useful against herpes infections.

Some researchers believe that if a virus is responsible for multiple sclerosis, it may be a common virus that causes no problems for most of the population, but may cause demyelination in a susceptible person. Some of the suspect viruses include the herpes simplex type 1 and the measles viruses. The herpes virus is the one that causes cold sores on the face, not the one that causes sores on the genitalia.

Despite frustrating dead ends in connecting multiple sclerosis to any specific virus, many bits of evidence do implicate the measles virus. The T lymphocytes in individuals with multiple sclerosis often exhibit an inappropriately vigorous reaction to the measles virus long after the person has had measles. This vigorous reaction is thought to indicate virus that is still in the body, and one of the body cells that might harbor the virus is the oligodendrocyte, the cell that makes myelin in the central nervous system. The autoimmune system might attack the oligodendrocytes in a misdirected effort to rid the body of measles virus. Part of the process in which the immune system attacks cells is by recognizing elements on their surfaces. Presumably people with certain *surface markers* on their oligodendrocytes, as these elements are called, are at greater risk for attack than those with markers that discourage attack. This could explain why certain classes of markers, called *HLA types,* are more likely targets.

If a virus is responsible for the disease, either directly or indirectly, one of the treatment options that becomes feasible is a vaccine. Recent research has suggested a link between an infection with a type of virus called a *retrovirus* and the abnormal immune activity typical of multiple sclerosis. One retrovirus that kills a class of white blood cells that is essential for immunity has already been identified. Attack by a similar virus might disable the immune system enough to allow the abnormal immune behavior typical of multiple sclerosis.

If a vaccine were developed against a virus important in the appearance of multiple sclerosis, people at high risk for developing the disease could be protected. This may be a complex task with retroviruses, however, because of variability in their protein structure. A uniform structure is vital to the development of an effective vaccine.

Prostaglandins

There has been some recent interest in the impact of manipulating various hormones and hormone-like factors in people with multiple sclerosis. One family of such hormone-like factors is the prostaglandin family. This family of substances plays a role in several different bodily systems including the blood-clotting system and the immune system. That any prostaglandins can affect the course of multiple sclerosis remains to be shown.

Aminopyridine

4-Aminopyridine and 3,4-diaminopyridine, two drugs administered by injection into veins, have been used for some people with multiple sclerosis, and the results have been encouraging. The rationale is that they alter conduction along nerves and may enable conduction to occur along demyelinated segments. The conduction is slower than normal, but enough of the information relayed by the nerve fibers is transmitted to improve performance. Major complications of these drugs include seizures and pins-and-needles sensations. These agents are not yet commercially available for use in people with multiple sclerosis.

Genetic Susceptibility

Studies of animals with experimental allergic encephalomyelitis, a disease that produces changes similar to those seen with MS, have shown that genes influence susceptibility. Genetic studies are now being conducted on people with multiple sclerosis to see if they show similar susceptibility factors. Several areas on different human chromosomes have shown an association with multiple sclerosis, but these may reflect ethnic origin rather than linkage to multiple sclerosis susceptibility genes. Gene regions most often associated with multiple sclerosis in patients in the United States are common in those people with Scandinavian ancestry. Even in a relatively small country like Italy, there is a lower risk for an individual with ancestors from the south of the country than for one with ancestors from the north. There is probably not a single gene or even a small collection of genes that make the development of MS in any individual inevitable, but vulnerability is almost certainly related to ethnic background.

The Future

Ideally, an infectious agent will be found to be responsible for multiple sclerosis, a vaccine will be developed, and the disease will be wiped out. Despite years of frustrating work, this still appears to be a real possibility. For people who already have the disease, an agent developed through research on cytokines, myelin proteins, autoantibodies, or other substances under investigation may provide relief from deterioration and allow recovery of nervous system function. Relief of symptoms will improve with advances in agents that speed conduction along demyelinated nerve tracts, in drugs that reduce spasticity, and in techniques that correct bladder, bowel, and sexual dysfunctions. The advances of recent years are grounds for considerable optimism. Solutions to the problems caused by multiple sclerosis and a technique that prevents multiple sclerosis from developing will be found. After years of frustration, what affects multiple sclerosis is becoming evident. Manipulation of the disease is practical. Eradication of the disease should soon be possible.

Recommended Reading

For those interested in more technical discussions of the topics raised in this book, the following books and articles are recommended.

General Information

Cook, S (ed): *Handbook of Multiple Sclerosis.* New York, Marcel Dekker, 1990.

Hallpike, JF, Adams, CWM, and Tourtellotte, WW (eds): *Multiple Sclerosis: Pathology, Diagnosis, and Management.* Baltimore, Williams & Wilkins, 1983.

Kalb, RC, and Scheinberg, LC (eds): *Multiple Sclerosis and the Family.* New York, Demos Publishers, 1992.

Kuroiwa, YM, and Kurland, LT (eds): *Multiple Sclerosis East and West.* Fukuoka, Japan, Kyushu University Press, 1982.

Matthews, WB, et al: *McAlpine's Multiple Sclerosis,* 2nd ed. New York, Churchill Livingstone, 1991.

Paty, DW, and Ebers, GC: *Multiple Sclerosis.* Philadelphia, F.A. Davis, in press.

Sibley, WA (ed): *Therapeutic Claims in Multiple Sclerosis,* ed 3. Demos Publications, New York, 1992.

Wolinsky, JS: Multiple sclerosis. In Appel, SH (ed): *Current Neurology.* Chicago, Mosby-Year Book, Inc., 1993, vol. 13: 167–207.

Bovine Myelin

Weiner, HL, Mackin, GA, Matsui, M, et al: Double-blind pilot trial of oral tolerization with myelin antigens in multiple sclerosis. *Science* 1993;259:1321–1324.

Copolymer-1

Bornstein, MB, Miller, A, Slagle, S, et al: A pilot trial of Cop-1 in exacerbating-remitting multiple sclerosis. *New England Journal of Medicine* 1987;317:408–414.

Corticosteroids

Beck, RW, Cleary, PA, Trobe, JD, et al: The effect of corticosteroids for acute optic neuritis on the subsequent development of multiple sclerosis. *New England Journal of Medicine* 1993;329: 1764–1769.

Myers, LW: Treatment of multiple sclerosis with ACTH and corticosteroids. In Rudick, RA, and Goodkin, DE (eds): *Treatment of multiple sclerosis: Trial design, results, and future perspectives.* Heidelberg, Germany, Springer-Verlag, 1992:135–156.

Shapiro, RT: *Symptom Management in Multiple Sclerosis,* ed 2. Demos Publications, New York, 1994.

Diagnosis

Lee, KH, Hashimoto, SA, Hooge, JP, et al: Magnetic resonance imaging of the head in the diagnosis of multiple sclerosis: A prospective 2-year follow-up with comparison of clinical evaluation, evoked potentials, oligoclonal banding, and CT. *Neurology* 1991;41:657–660.

Paty, DW, Asbury, AK, Herndin, RM, et al: Use of magnetic resonance imaging in the diagnosis of multiple sclerosis: Policy statement. *Neurology* 1986;36:1575.

Poser, C (ed): *Diagnosis of Multiple Sclerosis.* New York, Thieme-Stratton, 1984.

Rizzo, JF, III, and Lessell, S: Risk of developing multiple sclerosis after uncompli-cated optic neuritis: A long-term prospective study. *Neurology* 1988;38:185–190.

Thompson, AJ, Kermode, AG, Wicks, D, et al: Major differences in the dynamics of primary and secondary progressive multiple sclerosis. *Annals of Neurology* 1991;29:53–62.

Disability

Francis, DA: An assessment of disability rating scales used in multiple sclerosis. *Archives of Neurology* 1991;48:299–301.

Kurtzke, JF: Rating neurological impairment in multiple sclerosis: An expanded disability status scale (EDSS). *Neurology* 1983;33:1444–1452.

Emotional and Intellectual Disturbances

Beatty, WW, et al: Clinical and demographic predictors of cognitive performance in multiple sclerosis: Do diagnostic type, disease duration, and disability matter? *Archives of Neurology* 1990;47:305–309.

Peyser, JM, et al: Guidelines for neuropsychological research in multiple sclerosis. *Archives of Neurology* 1990;47:94–97.

Rao, SM, et al: Cognitive dysfunction in multiple sclerosis. I. Frequency, patterns, and prediction. *Neurology* 1991;41:685–691.

Rao, S: Cognitive function in multiple sclerosis. II. Impact on employment and social functioning. *Neurology* 1991;41:692–696.

Rabins, PV, et al: Structural brain correlates of emotional disorder in multiple sclerosis. *Brain* 1986;109:585–597.

Schiffer, RB, et al: Depressive episodes in patients with multiple sclerosis. *American Journal of Psychiatry* 1983;140:1498.

Epidemiology

Anderson, DW, et al: Revised estimate of the prevalence of multiple sclerosis in the United States. *Annals of Neurology* 1992;31:333–336.

Immunity

Goodin, DS: The use of immunosupressive agents in the treatment of multiple sclerosis: a critical review. *Neurology* 1991;41:980–985.

Powrie, F, and Coffman, RL: Cytokine regulation of T-cell function: Potential for therapeutic intervention. *Immunology Today* 1993;14:270–274.

Vitetta, ES, Thorpe, PE, and Uhr, JW: Immunotoxins: Magic bullets or misguided missiles? *Immunology Today* 1993;14:252–259.

Weiner, HL, and Hofler, DA: Immunotherapy of multiple sclerosis. *Annals of Neurology* 1988;23:211–222.

Waksman, BH, and Reynolds, WE: Multiple sclerosis is a disease of immune regulation. *Proceedings of the Society for Experimental Biology and Medicine* 1984;175:282.

Interferon

Arnason, BGW: Interferon beta in multiple sclerosis. *Neurology* 1993;43:641–643.

IFNB Multiple Sclerosis Study Group: Interferon beta-1b is effective in relapsing-remitting multiple sclerosis. I. Clinical results of a multicenter randomized, double-blind, placebo-controlled trial. *Neurology* 1993;43:655–661.

Jacobs, L, et al: Intrathecal interferon reduces exacerbations of multiple sclerosis. *Science* 1981;214:1026.

Panitch, HS, et al: Treatment of multiple sclerosis with gamma interferon: Exacerbations associated with activation of the immune system. *Neurology* 1987;37:1097–1102.

Paty, DW, Li, DKB, and UBC MS/MRI Study Group: Interferon beta-1b is effective in relapsing-remitting multiple sclerosis. II. MRI analysis results of a multicenter, randomized, double-blind, placebo-controlled trial. *Neurology* 1993;43:662–667.

Quality Standards Subcommittee of the American Academy of Neurology: Practice advisory on selection of patients with multiple sclerosis for treatment with Betaseron. *Neurology* 1994;44:1537–1540.

Rudick, RA: Betaseron for multiple sclerosis. Implications for therapeutics. *Archives of Neurology* 1994;51:125–128.

Magnetic Resonance Scanning

McFarlin, HF, et al: Using gadolinium enhanced MRI lesions to monitor disease activity in multiple sclerosis. *Annals of Neurology* 1992;32:758–766.

Paty, DW, McFarlin, DE, and McDonald, WI: Magnetic resonance imaging and laboratory aids in the diagnosis of multiple sclerosis. *Annals of Neurology* 1991;29:3–5.

Wiebe, S, Lee, DH, et al: Serial cranial and spinal cord magnetic resonance imaging in multiple sclerosis. *Annals of Neurology* 1991;32:643–650.

Mortality

Sadovnick, AD, et al: Cause of death in patients attending multiple sclerosis clinics. *Neurology* 1991;41:1193–1196.

Silberberg, DH, supplement editor: Multiple sclerosis: approaches to management. *Annals of Neurology* 1994, (suppl) 36.

Pregnancy

Birk, K, Ford, C, Smeltzer, S, Ryan, D, et al: The clinical course of multiple sclerosis during pregnancy and the puerperium. *Archives of Neurology* 1990,47:738–742.

Poser, S, and Poser, W: Multiple sclerosis and gestation. *Neurology* 1983;33:1422.

Thompson, D, et al: The effects of pregnancy in multiple sclerosis: A retrospective study. *Neurology* 1986;36:1097–1099.

Sexual Dysfunction

Schover, L, et al: Orgasm phase dysfunctions in multiple sclerosis. *Journal of Sex Research* 1988;24:548–554.

Lechtenberg, R, and Ohl, DA: *Sexual Dysfunction.* Philadelphia, Lea and Febiger, 1994.

Glossary of Terms

Acetylcholine. One of the chemicals used by nerves to communicate with each other.

ACTH (adrenocorticotropic hormone, ACTH, Duracton). A substance produced by the brain that regulates the production of steroids by the adrenal gland. This material can be produced artificially and is often used to manage flare-ups of multiple sclerosis.

Anesthesia. Loss of all pain and touch perception over part or all of the body.

Antibodies. Proteins produced by special cells in the immune system that attack germs, parasites, and other substances that do not belong in the body.

Ataxia. Poorly coordinated walking or other limb movements.

Autoantibodies. Proteins produced by the immune system that attach to and evoke an attack upon the individual's own tissue.

Autoimmune disease. A process in which the body's immune system causes illness by attacking elements, such as particular cells or materials, that are normal and essential for health.

Baclofen (Lioresal). An antispasticity agent presumed to interfere with spinal cord activity that produces abnormal muscle tone in the arms and legs.

B-cell. A type of white blood cell that matures into an antibody-producing cell when exposed to specific stimuli.

Betaseron. See Interferon beta-1b.

Bovine myelin. A form of myelin derived from cows and given by mouth. See Myelin.

Brain stem. The area of nerve cells and nerve fibers at the base of the brain that connects to the spinal cord but is still within the skull.

Brain-stem auditory evoked potential. Electrical impulses recorded from the base of the brain in response to repeated clicks.

Central nervous system. That part of the nervous system covered by the meninges and including the brain, spinal cord, and optic nerves.

Centrocecal scotoma. A blind spot that interferes with central vision.

Cerebellum. A part of the brain at the base of the skull that is responsible for many aspects of coordination.

Circumduction. A pattern of moving the legs, usually caused by partial paralysis or spasticity, that requires the person to swing the upper leg widely at the hip.

Clonus. Repeated contraction and relaxation of a muscle.

Colchicine. A drug (used for decades to treat gout) that some claim reduces the frequency and severity of flare-ups in multiple sclerosis.

Computed tomography. See CT scan.

Copolymer-1. A protein currently undergoing experimental tests for use in patients with relapsing-remitting multiple sclerosis.

Corticotropin. See ACTH.

Cortisone. A steroid hormone given to some people with multiple sclerosis to reduce acute inflammations in the nervous system.

CT scan. A computerized imaging system that uses X rays to determine the density of different spots in the body. By producing a map of the densities at thousands of spots in the brain, it discloses normal and abnormal structures.

Cytokine. A soluble agent produced primarily by cells of the immune system, which modulates the activity of various elements of the immune system as well elements outside the immune system.

Dantrolene sodium (Dantrium). An antispasticity agent.

Demyelination. The stripping off of the myelin lining of nerve fibers by a disease process.

Disuse atrophy. Loss of substance, as in the loss of bulk in a muscle that is used little or not at all.

Dysarthria. Problems with the clarity or rhythm of speech resulting from damage to the central or peripheral nervous system.

Dysesthesia. A painful alteration of touch and pressure perception.

Edema. Swelling in the brain or elsewhere caused by the abnormal accumulation of fluid.

Electroencephalography (EEG). A diagnostic technique that amplifies and records the normal electrical activity in the brain.

Evoked potentials. Electrical signals recorded from the central nervous system that appear in response to repetitive stimuli, such as a clicking noise, a flashing light, or an electrical shock.

Exacerbation. Acute worsening or flare-up of neurologic signs and symptoms, usually associated with inflammation and demyelination in the brain or spinal cord.

Fecal incontinence. Loss of control of bowel movements.

Flaccid bladder. An abnormally distensible urinary bladder, developing with decreased nervous system control of the muscles in the bladder walls.

Flare-up. See exacerbation.

Focal deficits. Impaired strength or sensation over a limited part of the body.

Footdrop. Impaired or absent ability to bend the foot upward at the ankle.

Gait ataxia. Broad-based, staggering patterns of walking caused by poor coordination.

Gamma globulin. A family of antibodies that is increased in the spinal fluid of many people with multiple sclerosis.

Hyperbaric oxygen therapy. A discredited treatment that uses oxygen under pressure to raise body tissue levels of oxygen.

Hyperpathia. A disturbance in which a patch of skin is uncomfortably sensitive to minor stimuli.

Immunoglobulin. A general term for the various types of antibodies produced by the immune system.

Impotence. Poor or absent erection of the penis. This is an obstacle to sexual intercourse for some men with multiple sclerosis.

Incidence. The proportion of a population affected by a disease or exhibiting a trait over a defined interval of time.

Incontinence. The inability to hold urine or stool until urination or defecation is intended.

Interferon. A class of substances produced by the body's immune system in response to certain viral infections.

Interferon alpha. A specific interferon that has been used in experimental studies and is alleged to reduce exacerbations and new lesions seen using MR imaging in people with relapsing-remitting multiple sclerosis.

Interferon beta-1a. A specific interferon, structurally similar to Interferon beta-1b, under development as an agent that might affect the course of MS in some individuals.

Interferon beta-1b (Betaseron). A specific interferon that has been approved for use in ambulatory individuals (those able to walk) with relapsing-remitting multiple sclerosis to reduce the frequency of exacerbations.

Interleukin. A family of substances affecting the immune system, which play an important role in inflammation and other aspects of immunity.

Intranuclear ophthalmoplegia. A disturbance of coordinated eye movements occuring when nystagmus develops in the eye directed inward when looking to the side but does not appear when the eye turns inward to focus on an approaching object.

Lhermitte's sign. Briskly flexing the neck forward may produce an electric sensation running down the spine or into the limbs in people with multiple sclerosis.

Lioresal. See baclofen.

Lymphocyte. A type of white blood cell of considerable importance in the immune system.

Macrophage. A scavenger cell involved in demyelination.

Magnetic resonance imaging (MRI, MR, NMR). A diagnostic technique that uses the properties of different substances in a magnetic field to produce images of the fine structure of the brain, spinal cord, and other parts of the body.

Megavitamins. A popular, but ineffective, therapeutic approach to MS involving high doses of multiple vitamins.

Methylprednisolone. A corticosteroid injected into veins to reduce the duration of MS flare-ups or to manage optic neuritis; it has been associated with a delay in the worsening of multiple sclerosis signs and symptoms if given when optic neuritis is the only apparent sign of disease.

MR, MRI. See magnetic resonance imaging.

Myelin. The fatty insulation of nerve fibers that is damaged in multiple sclerosis.

Myelin basic protein. A component of the spinal fluid that is increased in some people with multiple sclerosis.

Myelography. An X ray of the spinal cord in which a relatively opaque dye is injected into the cerebrospinal fluid. The dye flows into the space around the spinal cord and reveals irregularities or obstructions.

Nerve fibers. Extensions from the body of a nerve cell, capable of transmitting electrical pulses as part of the information handling by the nervous system.

Neuron. An individual nerve cell.

Neurologic disease. Any disorder of the nervous system.

Nuclear magnetic resonance (NMR). See magnetic resonance imaging.

Nystagmus. Rhythmical jerking movements of the eyes.

Oligoclonal banding. Accumulations in the spinal fluid of excessive amounts of limited classes of antibodies.

Oligodendrocytes. Cells in the brain and spinal cord that produce the myelin sheath that insulates nerve fibers.

Optic atrophy. Degeneration of the optic nerve.

Optic nerve. The bundle of nerve fibers formed by the light-sensitive retina of the eye that extends from the eyes and connects to the brain.

Optic neuritis. Inflammation of the optic nerve that causes temporary or permanent loss of vision and is often associated with pain in the eye at the time vision deteriorates.

Oxygen therapy. See hyperbaric oxygen therapy.

Paresthesias. Pins-and-needles sensations that develop when a pain pathway is damaged.

Peripheral nerve. A nerve outside the central nervous system.

Placebo effect. The apparently beneficial result of treatment that has no real value in the therapy of a medical problem. The apparent benefits occur because of the patient's expectation that the treatment will help.

Plaque. A patch of demyelinated or inflamed central nervous system tissue.

Plasma cells. Antibody-producing cells.

Prednisone (Apo-prednisone, Colisone, Deltasone, Paracort). A steroid drug related chemically and therapeutically to the steroid hormones normally made in the adrenal glands.

Prevalence. The proportion of the total population affected by a disease at one point in time.

Primrose oil. A source of essential fatty acids, advocated by some as an aid in the treatment of multiple sclerosis. It has no proven value as a treatment.

Remission. A decrease in the signs and symptoms of multiple sclerosis.

Retrograde ejaculation. Uncoordinated movement of semen along the ducts leading to the penis.

Scanning speech. A lilting or sing-song quality to speech that is exhibited in individuals with severe dysarthria.

Somatosensory evoked potentials. Electrical changes in the brain in response to repeated electrical shocks applied to a peripheral nerve.

Spasticity. Increased tone and resistance to movement developing in limb or trunk muscles because of damage in the central nervous system.

Synapse. The complex junction between nerve cells across which they communicate.

T cell. A type of white blood cell whose activities are influenced by the thymus gland.

Thymus. A small gland in the chest above the heart that influences the behavior of white blood cells and other elements of the body's immune system.

Tic douloureux. See trigeminal neuralgia.

Tone. The degree of tension (resistance to passive stretching) in a muscle.

Transverse myelitis. Inflammation in the spinal cord interfering with nerve function below the level of the inflammation.

Trigeminal neuralgia. Sharp, stabbing pain in the face that occasionally develops with multiple sclerosis.

Urinary retention. Involuntary accumulation of excessive urine in the bladder.

Vertigo. The illusion that the surroundings are spinning or moving. This sensation is usually accompanied by nausea and vomiting.

Visual evoked potential. An electrical response to repeated visual stimuli given as part of a diagnostic technique to detect optic neuritis.

Index

A "T" or an "F" following a page number indicates a table or a figure, respectively.